# Praise for *Listening In*

"*Listening In* is an invitation to slow down and tune into the quiet language of the body. With insight and compassion, Carrie DeJong demonstrates how reconnecting with internal sensations can support healing, regulation, and self-trust. This is a thoughtful and accessible guide for anyone interested in embodied, trauma-informed approaches to well-being."

—DR. ARIELLE SCHWARTZ, clinical psychologist, author of *The Complex PTSD Workbook* and *The Post-Traumatic Growth Guidebook*, and founder of the Center for Resilience Informed Therapy

"*Listening In* offers a timely and clinically grounded exploration of interoception as a foundational thread across trauma, mental health, and addiction. Carrie DeJong thoughtfully bridges neuroscience, somatic practice, and clinical insight in a way that is both accessible and practical for practitioners, while inviting general audiences to a clearer understanding of well-being, recovery, and the powerful connection between mind and body. This book makes an important contribution to how we understand regulation, recovery, and healing from the inside out."

—DR. CARSON McPHERSON, CEO of ROSC Solutions Group and adjunct professor at Simon Fraser University

"*Listening In* is an excellent, deeply researched, and accessible book about a critically important aspect of being alive and human. This book will absolutely change my approach to my own life and work. I can imagine returning to these insights often—and sharing them with those I support in their healing journeys."

—QUINCEY KIRSCHNER, executive director of Avalon Recovery Society, Vancouver, BC

"This book is not only for the curious psychotherapist. It provides a theoretical and scientific background for your work and very practical guidance for tackling clinical challenges. It introduces you to a perspective where psychological concepts are grounded in our felt senses, our actual lived experience, where mind and body are one. And if you are not a psychotherapist, you will learn about our felt senses and gain new insights."

—WOLF E. MEHLING, MD, professor emeritus at the University of California, San Francisco

# Listening In

## How Interoception Can Improve Your Mental and Emotional Health

**Carrie DeJong, RCC**

North Atlantic Books
Huichin, unceded Ohlone land
Berkeley, California

North Atlantic Books
An educational nonprofit organization
Huichin, unceded Ohlone land
2526 Martin Luther King Jr Way
Berkeley, CA 94704 USA
www.northatlanticbooks.com

Cover art © StudioM1 and filo via Getty Images
Cover design by Jess Morphew
Book design by Happenstance Type-O-Rama

Acquisitions editor: Francesca Walker • Production editor: Janelle Ludowise
Copyeditor: Swetha Rao • Proofreader: Chuck Hutchinson • Indexer: Ken DellaPenta

North Atlantic Books's publications are distributed to the US trade and internationally by Penguin Random House Publisher Services. For further information, visit our website at www.northatlanticbooks.com.

The authorized representative in the EU for product safety and compliance is Eucomply OÜ, Pärnu mnt 139b-14, 11317 Tallinn, Estonia, hello@eucompliancepartner.com, +33757690241.

Library of Congress Cataloging-in-Publication Data
Names: DeJong, Carrie author
Title: Listening in : how interoception can improve your mental and emotional health / Carrie DeJong.
Description: Berkeley, California : North Atlantic Books, [2026] | Includes bibliographical references and index. | Summary: "A guide to the interoceptive sensory system"— Provided by publisher.
Identifiers: LCCN 2026021045 (print) | LCCN 2026021046 (ebook) | ISBN 9798889843764 trade paperback | ISBN 9798889843771 ebook
Subjects: LCSH: Interoception | Senses and sensation | Mental health
Classification: LCC QP431 .D295 2026 (print) | LCC QP431 (ebook)
LC record available at https://lccn.loc.gov/2026021045
LC ebook record available at https://lccn.loc.gov/2026021046

1 2 3 4 5 6 7 8 9 MARQUIS 31 30 29 28 27 26

Printed in Canada

# Contents

PREFACE. . . . . vii

**Part One**
AN OVERVIEW OF INTEROCEPTION

1 Understanding Interoception . . . . . 3
2 The Science of Interoception . . . . . 13
3 Interoception in Daily Life . . . . . 23
4 How Interoception Is Measured . . . . . 35

**Part Two**
WHAT SHAPES OUR INTEROCEPTIVE EXPERIENCES

5 Miscommunication Between Body and Brain . . . . . 49
6 How Thoughts Shape Interoception . . . . . 57
7 The Influence of Early Attachments . . . . . 67
8 Understanding the Stress Response . . . . . 75
9 Trauma Symptoms and Interoceptive Interruptions . . . . . 85
10 Trauma and the Disrupted Sense of Self . . . . . 97

**Part Three**
CHALLENGES WITH INTEROCEPTION

11 Common Threads, Synergistic Impacts, and Unintended Consequences . . . . . 109
12 Anxiety Disorders . . . . . 119
13 Depression . . . . . 129
14 OCD and Related Disorders . . . . . 141
15 Substance Use and Addiction Disorders . . . . . 151

16 Disordered Eating . . . . . . . . . . . . . . . . . . . . . . . . . . 161
17 Neurodivergent Conditions . . . . . . . . . . . . . . . . . . . . . . 169
18 Physical Health . . . . . . . . . . . . . . . . . . . . . . . . . . . 179
19 Interpersonal Connections . . . . . . . . . . . . . . . . . . . . . . 191

**Part Four**
WHAT WORKS

20 Determining What's Helpful . . . . . . . . . . . . . . . . . . . . . 203
21 Individual Practices . . . . . . . . . . . . . . . . . . . . . . . . 217
22 Practitioner-Led Therapies and Approaches . . . . . . . . . . . . 229
23 What Comes Next? . . . . . . . . . . . . . . . . . . . . . . . . . 243

NOTES . . . . . . . . . . . . . . . . . . . . . . . . . . . . . . . . 245
INDEX . . . . . . . . . . . . . . . . . . . . . . . . . . . . . . . . 267
ACKNOWLEDGMENTS . . . . . . . . . . . . . . . . . . . . . . . . . . 277
ABOUT THE AUTHOR . . . . . . . . . . . . . . . . . . . . . . . . . 279

# Preface

*Interoception* is a fundamental part of our lives, yet many people know very little about it. I'm on a mission to change that, because this internal sense plays a crucial role in our well-being. The simplest way to understand it is to recognize that it functions as one of our sensory systems. Just as sight, taste, and touch inform us about the world around us, interoception informs us about what is happening inside our bodies.

Some interoceptive signals are easy to identify—hunger, thirst, or the need to empty the bladder. But interoception extends far beyond these basics. It provides essential information that shapes our physical health, emotional states, decision-making, and sense of self. Interoceptive awareness offers a powerful lens for understanding many of the challenges people face today, including anxiety, depression, addiction, trauma, chronic pain, and relationship issues.

A few years ago, I delivered a TEDx talk on interoception, centered around the theme "clarity." Preparing that talk deepened my interest in this often-overlooked sensory system and its relevance to nearly every aspect of human functioning. It also heightened my awareness of how rarely interoception is discussed outside academic and clinical settings, despite its profound importance.

As a therapist, I support individuals who have experienced trauma, chronic stress, and addiction. My approach is grounded in an understanding of how the nervous system works and in recognizing that symptoms are often adaptive responses to overwhelm, not personal failures. Over the past fifteen years, I have developed a deep interest in neurobiology and body-centered therapy, especially in helping people understand how their nervous system influences their thoughts, emotions, and behaviors. I enjoy making complex neuroscience accessible and useful, even for those without a background in the field.

*Listening In* is my effort to make interoception understandable, practical, and relevant to everyday life. What follows is an invitation to deepen your connection with your body—to notice its signals, understand what they communicate, and learn to respond with greater clarity and care. I hope this book helps you experience your inner sensations not as something to control or ignore, but as meaningful information that can guide you toward greater health, resilience, and well-being.

# Part One

# AN OVERVIEW OF INTEROCEPTION

# 1

# Understanding Interoception

Have you ever watched one of those YouTube compilations where toddlers get their first pair of glasses? The glasses are new and uncomfortable, and the toddlers can be a little fussy at first. Some even try to remove them. Then it happens: They see clearly for the first time in their lives, and everything changes. The fussing stops. Their eyes widen in amazement. They begin to look around in wonder. A huge smile spreads across their face as they see their parents and the world around them in a completely new and exciting way. I find it incredibly heartwarming!

Compare this to video compilations of individuals hearing for the first time after receiving cochlear implants, which show mixed results. While some people are clearly delighted, others seem overwhelmed by the sounds they hear. Their own voices feel strange and uncomfortable to them. Often, there are tears—some of joy, and for others tears that signal a distinct unease with this sudden entry into the world of sound.

I use these two illustrations to highlight a point about interoception, one of our eight sensory systems. The other seven are sight, hearing, smell, taste, touch, the vestibular system (balance), and proprioception (movement). Interoception is not as well known or as widely understood as our other senses, such as sight or hearing, but it is an essential part of our existence. Some individuals experience interoception differently than others, much like the significant variations in our ability to see or hear.

Learning more about interoception can be like seeing clearly for the first time with glasses or hearing for the first time with cochlear implants. The experience can produce mixed results, depending on the individual. For some, enhancing awareness of bodily signals and understanding their meanings can be a positive and enriching process. For others, it may feel uncomfortable, especially if they've never considered their inner sensations and the messages those sensations convey. Yet interoception can reveal a whole new world. I believe that looking at ourselves through the lens of our interoceptive experiences helps us better understand ourselves and our challenges and moves us toward greater wellness.

## A Brief History of Interoception

Interoception is essentially our sense of internal perception. Charles S. Sherrington, a British neurophysiologist, coined the term *interoceptive* in 1906, giving the concept its original meaning. Sherrington used it to describe the sensations we experience from our digestive system. The term *interoception* itself was not introduced until the 1940s.[1] By then, it had expanded to include sensations from the lungs, heart, and urinary tract.

Still, that wasn't the first time researchers made reference to bodily sensations or the role they play. In the late 1800s, scientists William James and Carl Lange suggested that emotions arise from physical sensations. They proposed that we don't have a bodily reaction (like trembling) because we're afraid; rather, we feel afraid because we notice ourselves trembling.[2] In other words, emotional experiences don't start in our brains but in our bodies. More recent research, such as the work of Bechara and Damasio, highlights how physical sensations shape our emotional lives.[3] These scientists generally agree that emotions result from bodily sensations that the mind works to make sense of. Interoception is essential in this process.

As neuroscience has evolved over the past century, so too has the definition of interoception. Beyond basic bodily sensations, such as sensing our heartbeat or feeling a full bladder, interoception now encompasses internal cues including hunger, thirst, fatigue, and fluctuations in body temperature. It also includes pain signals that originate internally, from our skin and even our teeth.[4] We now understand that internal cues are involved in our emotional processes. All these sensations reflect interoception at work. Yet interoception is a far more complex process than merely sensing what occurs in our bodies; it also involves how the brain interprets and integrates these signals.

## The Role of Interoceptive Messages

Bodily sensations occur all the time. Sometimes we are aware of them, such as when our hearts beat faster from exercise or when we shiver from the cold. At other times, we may be able to bring our awareness to sensations that are always happening but that we're not necessarily noticing, such as when our chest expands as we take a deep breath. Even though we're always breathing, we typically don't notice what it *feels* like. We may take these sensations for granted, yet they are essential to our physical well-being.

These interoceptive messages convey crucial information about our body's condition and the management of bodily needs, such as food, water, air, or medical attention. When you attempt to hold your breath, your body sends strong interoceptive signals indicating that you need air. Your heart rate decreases, you begin to feel dizzy, and you experience an intense urge to breathe. This is your body's way of signaling that you require oxygen. Hunger pangs signal the need for nourishment. Fatigue cues the need for rest. Interoceptive sensations or messages clearly play an essential role in managing all our bodily needs.

Just as interoceptive messages inform us about the body's physical state, affective interoceptive messages help us sense how those bodily states feel. These messages arise when the brain interprets internal sensations and assigns them emotional meaning.[5] They help us notice what feels comfortable, uncomfortable, or in need of care. For example, stepping outside on a cold day may cause shivering—a clear signal that the body is cooling down. If you dislike being cold, the discomfort from that sensation encourages you to put on a coat. Conversely, stepping into an air-conditioned building on a hot summer day may feel pleasant and relieving, even though the body still responds to the temperature change. In each case, sensation and feeling work together to guide behavior.

Pleasant affective sensations often show up as ease or comfort—feeling pleasantly full after a meal or invigorated after a walk. Unpleasant sensations, on the other hand, signal tension, distress, or unmet needs, such as the discomfort of hunger or thirst. Alongside physical interoceptive signals, these affective cues support everyday regulation and well-being. Many operate outside conscious awareness, quietly shaping our mood, decisions, and emotional responses.

To sum up, affective interoceptive messages extend the role of interoception beyond the bodily cues necessary for our physical survival. They help shape emotional experiences, guide daily choices, and influence motivation in subtle yet powerful ways—reflecting what researchers such as Damasio describe as the central role of bodily sensations in emotion, motivation, and everyday decision-making.

## Interoception: A Two-Way Street

Interoception is not just about sensing bodily sensations—it also involves the brain's ability to receive, interpret, and respond to these signals. It is a bidirectional process, meaning that the body sends messages to the brain, and the brain sends messages back to the body. This dynamic feedback loop helps regulate and manage our bodily functions. Interoceptive cues from the body are crucial signals that inform the brain about what's happening, such as pain or stressors. The brain processes these signals and responds by adjusting the system—by increasing heart rate, releasing stress hormones, or doing whatever the body needs at that moment.

Sometimes, communication between the brain and body occurs in ways we aren't consciously aware of, such as regulating blood sugar levels. We don't have to consciously choose to sweat to cool down on a hot day. At other times, interoceptive sensations act as signals that prompt us to take necessary action, like drinking water when thirsty or napping when we're tired.

This bidirectional process is unique to each of us, shaped by how we individually interpret or understand our bodily sensations. We can assign different emotional or physical meanings to the sensations our bodies produce. For instance, people may interpret an elevated heart rate while climbing stairs in many ways. One might perceive it as anxiety, another might attribute it to being out of shape, while yet another might worry that it signals a heart attack. How we evaluate or interpret our sensations greatly influences our responses to them and has significant implications for our well-being. Interoception isn't only about our internal sensations; it's about how we respond to them.

It is also important to recognize that these responses are shaped by our lived experiences. Throughout this book, we will explore how trauma, racism, poverty, family separation, and chronic stress can affect how comfortable we feel in our bodies and how easily we stay connected to what we sense inside. In this way, interoception is not just biological—it is also deeply relational and shaped by context, reflecting both the challenges we've faced and the support and resources available to us.

Because interoception plays such an essential role in well-being, it makes sense that difficulties with it would be present in people experiencing health and mental health challenges. Research has found that problems with interoception are linked to mental health issues, including depression, anxiety, obsessive-compulsive disorder (OCD), addiction disorders, eating disorders, suicidality, and post-traumatic stress disorder (PTSD). Interoceptive difficulties also contribute to physical conditions such as fibromyalgia, irritable bowel syndrome (IBS), and chronic pain.[6] While a well-functioning interoceptive system supports overall well-being, those who struggle with interoception often face significant challenges in daily life.

## Why Interoception? Why Now?

Although interoception may not be widely recognized, the concept itself is familiar. Over recent decades, interest in body awareness, "gut feelings," and the mind–body connection has steadily grown. Research on the vagus nerve has further highlighted the body's role in physical and mental well-being.

We can track the evolution of psychotherapy over the past 140 years to better understand why there is so much interest in the mind–body connection today. In the mid-twentieth century, behavioral therapy emerged, focusing on helping individuals *unlearn* behaviors that contributed to mental and physical health issues. This evolved into cognitive behavioral therapy (CBT) in the 1960s, a treatment that remains widely used today.

By the 1970s, clinicians increasingly recognized that therapeutic change requires not only cognitive insight but also awareness and regulation of bodily signals. Earlier pioneers such as F. M. Alexander and Moshé Feldenkrais had already shown how movement and posture shape psychological experience. Building on this work, Peter Levine later developed Somatic Experiencing, emphasizing sensation-based approaches to trauma recovery. During this period, Ron Kurtz introduced Hakomi, a body-centered psychotherapy aimed at transforming unconscious beliefs through experiential awareness. In the 1980s, acceptance-based therapies such as acceptance and commitment therapy (ACT) and mindfulness-based cognitive therapy (MBCT) expanded CBT by integrating mindfulness, acceptance, and compassion. Jon Kabat-Zinn's development of Mindfulness-Based Stress Reduction (MBSR) played a key role in shaping today's mindfulness practices.

Body-based therapy tools have become increasingly mainstream. Additional somatic methods, including Sensorimotor Psychotherapy and trauma-informed yoga, have been developed. Today, techniques like grounding, breathwork, movement, and touch are common in psychotherapy. These approaches have helped shift the field toward a more integrated, somatic-based understanding of how the mind and body work together to promote healing.

The study of interoception has experienced significant growth in recent years, partly because body–brain science has shifted from being viewed as unconventional or even strange to being widely accepted as central to understanding human experience. We've come to realize that we are not just brains with bodies—our body and brain are deeply interconnected, influencing nearly every aspect of our lives. The rising emphasis on whole-person wellness has also contributed to this shift. Interoception supports physical, mental, emotional, and social well-being—it is essential to all these dimensions of who we are.

We also need to rethink how mental health is evaluated and treated. Many approaches emphasize symptoms and diagnoses without fully investigating their underlying factors. Psychological and therapeutic treatments often target visible signs—such as anxiety, low mood, overeating, or inattention—but may miss the root causes beneath. As I often say, "The problem is the problem." Treating symptoms alone can provide short-term relief, but true healing requires understanding what truly drives them.

Research increasingly shows that disrupted interoception is a key factor in many physical and mental health concerns.[7] Exposure to chronic stress—such as racism, poverty, trauma, and chronic adversity—often disrupts interoception because survival sometimes requires ignoring or distrusting bodily signals. This makes interoception a powerful framework for understanding not just what is happening, but why. Moving beyond symptom-focused approaches, interoception provides a pathway for both healing and prevention. In the chapters ahead, we'll examine trauma more closely, including the Adverse Childhood Experiences (ACE) Study, and discuss how reconnecting with the body supports long-term well-being.

## What Shapes My Perspective

My work as a therapist has been shaped by a long-standing curiosity about the mind–body connection and its role in healing. Early in my career, while working in a trauma program for children and teens, I was introduced to somatic therapy. Its focus on the nervous system's response to trauma immediately resonated with me, revealing the profound wisdom held in the body—and how traumatic experiences can disrupt our ability to interpret internal signals accurately.

This early exposure shifted the way I understood symptoms. Rather than seeing anxiety, shutdown, or emotional reactivity as problems to eliminate, I began to see them as meaningful responses shaped by the nervous system's attempts to protect. Somatic therapy offered a framework for helping people reconnect with their internal experience in ways that felt safer, clearer, and more compassionate.

Further study of autonomic regulation deepened this understanding. I came to appreciate more fully how shifts in physiological state influence our sense of safety, emotional patterns, and capacity for connection. This continues to shape how I support clients in noticing internal cues, settling their nervous systems, and approaching their experiences with curiosity and self-compassion.

This blend of clinical experience, somatic training, and neurobiological research forms the foundation of this book. Throughout these chapters, I offer clear explanations, research-based insights, and practical guidance drawn from decades of therapeutic work. But this book does more than explain interoception—it invites you to practice it. You'll find reflective questions, simple exercises, and clinical illustrations that demonstrate the many ways *listening in* can unfold.

Because people approach learning and well-being differently, this book is intentionally both scientific and experiential. You'll gain a solid understanding of how interoception works while also being encouraged to explore your own internal experience in ways that feel accessible and meaningful.

Ultimately, this book invites you to deepen your relationship with your body—to listen to its messages, understand how your nervous system shapes your thoughts and emotions, and discover how interoception can support healing and emotional well-being. It is a privilege to share this journey with you as we explore the ongoing dialogue between body and mind.

## Meet Our Clients

To help illustrate what interoception looks like in everyday life, I've included some "case studies." While these scenarios aren't based on actual people, they reflect common experiences that show how interoception influences our daily lives. Their stories—their struggles with emotional regulation and mental health, and their personal experiences of interoception—are typical of many of my clients.

*Roland is an almost-retired accountant with grown children and a failing marriage. His wife says he is emotionally distant and unable to connect with her or their adult children. Work is his main focus. Roland reports no significant emotional distress despite his marital struggles.*

*Catherine is a forty-five-year-old nurse, married with three school-aged children. To others, her life looks successful—her home is a hub for family gatherings, and she appears highly capable. Yet underneath that image, she relentlessly pushes herself to meet her own high standards.*

*Ava is nineteen and aspires to be a famous fashion influencer. She spends her time creating content for her social media accounts. Her feeds are filled with highly edited selfies and carefully staged shots featuring her latest clothes, jewelry, and luxury items—many of which are gifts from the wealthy men she dates. To maintain her ideal image, she frequently restricts food and overexercises.*

*Jason is a thirty-three-year-old construction worker who is currently single. He has a five-year-old son with whom he has no contact after the child's mother charged him with assault following an alcohol-fueled argument. Jason acknowledges that his quick temper creates problems for him, but he often blames others for his actions.*

*Lauren is a thirty-five-year-old preschool teacher who lives alone and is deeply committed to her work with children. She is often described as nurturing, compassionate, and exceptionally attuned to others' emotions. While her sensitivity helps her care deeply, it often comes at the cost of her own emotional and physical well-being.*

*Hailey is twenty-five and struggles with health anxiety. Ongoing fear and preoccupation with the possibility of getting sick dominate her daily life. She often worries about germs and contamination and repeatedly seeks reassurance from her doctor, despite being told she is healthy. Her intense anxiety and panic attacks make it hard for her to feel confident managing everyday activities.*

*David is a thirty-nine-year-old business owner whose life unraveled after betrayal by a former business partner, leaving him depressed and withdrawn. He now struggles to connect with his wife, his twin sons, and the hobbies he once loved. His conflict avoidance has hurt both his business and his marriage, deepening his sense of being stuck. At his core, David feels like a failure—a belief that shapes his relationships and choices.*

As you journey through this book, you'll meet these individuals multiple times. They're here to help you better understand how interoception shows up in everyday experiences and to illustrate how people perceive bodily sensations differently, leading to different outcomes. You'll also see how interoceptive challenges contribute to mental health issues.

## Where We're Going

This book is organized into four parts that explore key aspects of interoception, highlighting its significance in daily life and its effects on both physical and mental health.

Part 1 explains interoception and its importance for well-being. It examines how awareness of internal body signals helps regulate the body, shape emotional experiences, support clear thinking, and enhance our sense of self and connection with others. Research also shows that many mental health challenges are linked to disruptions in interoception. Chapter 2 focuses on the role of interoception in mental health and provides a solid scientific foundation for the rest of the book.

Part 2 looks at the differences in how people experience interoception and the factors that influence how individuals perceive and interpret their internal sensations, including early attachment patterns and traumatic experiences.

Part 3 examines how interoceptive disturbances are connected to various mental health disorders, including anxiety, depression, PTSD, addiction, and chronic pain. It highlights how interoceptive challenges vary in their contributions to, and manifestations within, each of these disorders.

Part 4 identifies the resources and tools that help cultivate healthy interoceptive awareness. No book about interoception would be complete without offering ways to nurture a deeper connection to the signals our bodies send.

# 2

# The Science of Interoception

Interoception is interesting in part because of its complexity. Several bodily processes work together to enable us to sense, interpret, and regulate the signals coming from our body.

Consider the different bodily systems listed next, all of which send interoceptive signals.[1] As you read through this list, take a moment to notice which of these signals you are aware of in this moment or have experienced at another time.

**Cardiovascular system.** You might notice sensations from your heart and blood vessels, such as your heart beating, palpitations, or blood-pressure changes.

- Can you feel your heartbeat right now?
- Are you more aware of it when you're physically exerting yourself?
- Do you notice your heart beating more when you are anxious or stressed?

**Respiratory system.** Your lungs, airways, and breathing muscles send signals about your breath rate, the effort needed to breathe, and oxygen levels.

- Can you bring attention to your breath and notice what it feels like to breathe?
- What sensation changes do you notice if you hold your breath for ten to fifteen seconds?
- Can you feel different parts of your chest and abdomen expand when you take a deep breath?

**Gastrointestinal system.** The stomach and intestines produce sensations like hunger, fullness, nausea, digestive discomfort, and the urge to defecate.

- How easily can you sense hunger signals?
- Can you notice the difference between being pleasantly full and too full?
- Can you tell the difference between hunger signals and how stress or anxiety affects your stomach?

**Urinary system.** Signals from the kidneys and bladder indicate when the bladder is full and the need to urinate.

- Can you tell how full your bladder feels?
- Do you notice differences in the sense of urgency?
- Can you hold your bladder, or do you need to empty it immediately?

**Nociceptive (pain) system.** This system transmits pain signals from your tissues and organs, and it can also sense itchiness.

- Is your pain tolerance high or low?
- Can you describe a pain you're feeling (e.g., is it sharp, dull, throbbing)?
- Are you able to rate your level of pain on a scale of 1–10?

**Thermoregulatory system.** Your body monitors both internal and external temperatures, helping you sense warmth, cold, and temperature changes.

- Are you feeling warm, cold, or just right in this moment?
- Can you feel the difference in temperature in your nostrils depending on whether you are inhaling or exhaling?
- Can you notice your hands become warm when you rub them together?

**Endocrine (hormonal) system.** Hormones like melatonin, which makes you sleepy, and adrenaline, which is part of our stress response, generate interoceptive signals.

- What bodily sensations do you experience when you're sleepy?
- What shifts occur in your body when you're stressed?
- Have you ever noticed sensations of shakiness related to low blood sugar?

**Immune system.** It communicates through signals such as inflammation, fatigue, and fever.

- Can you recall some of the sensations you experienced the last time you had a fever or felt sick?
- What symptoms do you experience if you have an allergic reaction to something?
- Are you usually aware of inflammation, warmth, or throbbing that occurs with an injury such as a bruise or a small cut?

Beyond these bodily systems, interoceptive signals are also detected and interpreted by specialized sensors called interoceptors. Mechanoreceptors are one such type of interoceptor; they detect mechanical forces like stretch or pressure within your organs, muscles, and joints.

- Take a moment to notice the sensations of your chest muscles expanding and contracting with each breath.
- Can you remember a time when you ate too much and felt uncomfortable?
- Have you ever been aware of your heart beating or felt your pulse without trying to?

I hope this discussion and the accompanying questions encourage you to explore more of your own experiences with interoceptive sensations. They are constantly happening, and, as we've come to understand, our ability to notice and understand them is essential for our well-being.

## The Vagus Nerve: Our Interoceptive Superhighway

Interoception involves how we interpret signals from sensors in our organs, muscles, skin, and blood vessels. These sensors detect changes such as pressure, temperature, and chemical levels, then send this information to the brain via autonomic and sensory pathways. Much of this process happens automatically, shaping how we feel long before we can identify what is happening.

One of the key components in this process is the vagus nerve, which helps connect bodily sensations with our awareness of them. The vagus nerve is a two-way communication pathway that carries information between the brain and the body, helping the nervous system adjust to changing internal and external demands.[2] Its name comes from the Latin word *vagus*, meaning "wandering," a reference to its extensive reach throughout the body. The vagus nerve is actually a pair of nerves that originate in the brainstem and travel down the neck, linking the brain to organs such as the heart, lungs, stomach, and intestines.[3]

A large portion of vagal signals travel from the body to the brain, making the vagus nerve primarily a sensory pathway. Its central role is to keep the brain informed about what is happening inside the body, delivering continuous updates that help regulate vital functions like heart rate and blood pressure.[4]

The vagus nerve also plays a major role in the parasympathetic nervous system—the "rest and digest" branch that promotes relaxation, digestion, and recovery from stress. It is a key part of the gut–brain connection, which is increasingly recognized as vital for emotional regulation. When this pathway becomes disrupted, both physical and mental health can be affected.[5]

## The Insular Cortex

The vagus nerve and other neural pathways send signals to the *insular cortex*, also known as the insula, a part of the cerebral cortex located deep within the brain and a key hub for interoception. The insula helps the brain receive and interpret information from within the body—signals related to basic functions like breathing, heartbeat, pain, temperature, hunger, and the body's stress response.[6] But the insula does more than monitor the body; it also helps create emotional experiences.

Neuroscientist Bud Craig explains that emotions begin as physical sensations that the insula organizes and brings into awareness. In this way, the insula serves as a bridge between what the body senses and what we consciously feel as emotion.[7]

Craig also highlights the insula's role in shaping our sense of self. He notes that the anterior insular cortex (AIC) is activated across a wide range of experiences, including bodily sensations, emotions, self-recognition, attention, decision-making, perception, and even our sense of time. Since no other brain region participates in such a broad range of activities, Craig proposes that the AIC may be the generator of our moment-to-moment awareness.[8]

Craig explains that the insula is "crucial not only for emotional awareness but also for mental illness," noting that "distorted feelings produce mental illness."[9] Research echoes this idea: Changes in the insula are found across many conditions, including chronic pain, anxiety, depression, disordered eating, and addiction.[10] These are conditions in which internal signals become harder to interpret, tolerate, or trust. As we move through later chapters, we'll explore how interoception and the insula may shape, and be shaped by, various mental health challenges.

## Autonomic Regulation: Rest, Mobilization, and Recovery

The autonomic nervous system (ANS) is the part of the nervous system that operates automatically in the background. It controls breathing, heart rate, digestion, energy levels, and stress responses without us having to think about it—often before we even realize what we're feeling. It is commonly described as having two main branches:

- The sympathetic nervous system, which prepares the body for action.
- The parasympathetic nervous system, which supports rest, digestion, and recovery.

In daily life, we constantly switch between these two branches. The nervous system adjusts based on what we sense—both inside and outside—and these changes influence how we feel, think, and respond. These shifts can happen quickly, sometimes within seconds, and often occur before we consciously notice what has changed.

Different models describe autonomic regulation in various ways, but they generally agree on one key point: The nervous system is built to change its state in response to the situation, and these changes serve a protective purpose.

**Rest and recovery.** When the body perceives enough safety and support, parasympathetic activity helps the system recover. Breathing becomes more efficient, digestion improves, heart rate stabilizes, and the body can heal. This is the state most associated with rest, calmness, and emotional clarity.

You might notice it after a warm meal, when your body naturally shifts into digestion and repair, or when you sit down with a hot drink and feel your shoulders relax. Sometimes it arrives at the end of the day—getting into bed, exhaling more deeply, and realizing your mind is finally slowing down.

**Mobilization and action.** When the nervous system detects danger, whether real or perceived, it shifts toward sympathetic activation. Heart rate rises, breathing quickens, and attention narrows. This activated state is meant to help us respond quickly and effectively to any stressor our system perceives.[11]

You can feel it when you're running late and stuck behind a slow driver, when you walk into a room and realize you don't know anyone, or when you see an email with an urgent subject line and your body tenses before you've even read it. This is not a sign of dysfunction; it's a protective response.

**Flexibility as the goal.** Importantly, neither the rest state nor the mobilization state is the problem. The nervous system is meant to move and adapt. The goal isn't to be calm all the time—it's to have enough flexibility to mobilize when needed and to return to rest once the moment has passed.[12]

**Not everything fits fight-or-flight.** Flexibility also includes recognizing that the nervous system doesn't only switch between rest and action. Many people are familiar with fight-or-flight, but the nervous system has other protective responses as well. When danger feels intense, overwhelming, or impossible to respond to, the body may shift into states of immobilization.[13]

Some people experience this as freezing—a feeling of being stuck, unable to speak or move, even though they want to. This can happen during everyday moments, like going blank in the middle of a difficult conversation, being unable to find words during conflict, or feeling suddenly unable to act even though part of you knows you want to *do something.*

Others describe a deeper shutdown, where energy decreases, emotions go numb, or the world feels far away. This might look like feeling flat or disconnected after a stressful interaction, struggling to care about things you normally value, or wanting to withdraw and disappear even when nothing seems wrong on the surface. Dissociation is another experience that can occur in these states, such as feeling detached from the body or as if life is happening from afar.

These responses are not choices, nor do they indicate weakness. They are deeply biological strategies meant to help the system endure what feels overwhelming. The issue isn't that the nervous system experiences these states; it's getting stuck in them.

## Why Autonomic Regulation Matters for Interoception

Autonomic regulation is important for interoception because it influences how clearly we can sense, interpret, and trust what our body is telling us.

The same sensation can feel very different depending on whether the nervous system is calm, active, or shut down.

When the nervous system is flexible, internal cues tend to feel more coherent and easier to interpret. Sensations such as hunger, fatigue, tension, emotion, or the need for rest are more likely to register in a way that makes sense. It becomes easier to notice what you feel and respond with care.

When the nervous system becomes stuck in a high-activation state, internal sensations can feel intense, urgent, or overwhelming. People may experience overwhelming anxiety-like sensations—tightness in the chest, racing thoughts, agitation, nausea, or pain. In these moments, it can be difficult to distinguish between what the body is signaling and what the system is preparing for.

When the nervous system shifts into shutdown, signals can become muted or distant. Hunger, emotion, pain, and even the sense of being present in the body may fade into the background. People often describe feeling numb, foggy, or unsure of what they feel. In other words, interoception is not only about noticing sensations. It also involves recognizing the state of the nervous system when sensations arise, and how that state influences what we're feeling.

## Top-Down or Bottom-Up?

Earlier, we described interoception as a two-way connection between the body and the brain. But what does that actually mean? For a long time, interoception was viewed mainly as a one-way pathway: signals traveling from the body to the brain to help regulate basic functions that keep us alive. Much of this occurs automatically. We don't need to remember to breathe, digest food, or adjust our blood pressure.

We now understand something more nuanced. The brain doesn't simply receive body signals—it interprets them and responds. Interoception is less like a one-way message and more like a conversation: The body sends information upward, and the brain constantly sends signals back down. In simple terms, bottom-up signals carry information from the body to the brain. Top-down processes describe how the brain makes sense of those signals—and how it influences what we notice, how we interpret it, and what happens next.

### *Bottom-Up Signals: Messages from the Body*

Bottom-up signals are messages sent from the body to the brain. They travel through the vagus nerve and other pathways, relaying information about internal conditions. Most of this communication happens outside of awareness. But we tend to notice body signals when something changes or needs attention, such as our heart pounding after exercise, shivering in the cold, or hunger reminding us to eat.

These signals don't only relate to physical needs; they also shape our emotional world. Sensations and emotions often arrive together: Tightness in the chest can accompany worry, warmth can accompany affection, and a heavy stomach can accompany sadness. Emotions are not just thoughts; they are felt experiences rooted in the body.

### *Top-Down Processes: How the Brain Shapes What We Feel*

Top-down processes describe how the brain responds to bodily signals. Some responses happen automatically, while others require conscious awareness. Top-down processes help us

**Respond to needs.** We feel thirst, hunger, fatigue, or pain—and we decide how to respond.

**Decide what to pay attention to.** For example, we can notice our hunger but choose to delay eating until a stressful situation is resolved.

**Make meaning.** Is that sensation of warmth the result of exercise, a temperature change, or a fever?

**Recognize and regulate emotion.** The brain helps us identify what we're feeling and choose ways to take care of ourselves when emotions are strong.

**Build a sense of self.** Interoception helps create that felt sense of *me*, the continuous experience of being a person in a body. This sense of self is closely connected to the insular cortex, one of the brain's main interoceptive centers.

## Predictive Processing: The Brain as a Forecaster

Another piece of the puzzle is predictive processing. Rather than simply reacting to events as they occur, the brain constantly uses past experience to anticipate what is likely to happen next and prepare the body for it.[14]

In interoception, the brain continually predicts the signals it expects to receive from the body and compares those predictions with incoming signals. This ongoing process shapes our internal experience. When the brain's expectations align with the body's signals, sensations tend to feel clear and familiar. When they don't align, the mismatch often brings the body more clearly into awareness—sometimes as discomfort, uncertainty, or intensity—until the brain updates its expectations.

Pavlov's dogs offer a familiar example of how this process works. The dogs learned to salivate at the sound of a bell, because their brains predicted food was coming. When the bell no longer signaled food, the dogs gradually stopped salivating as their brains updated their expectations. Interoception works similarly. The brain constantly makes educated guesses about what's happening inside the body based on past experience—and revises those guesses when new information doesn't match.

This is also why thirst often fades almost immediately after drinking water, even though hydration takes time. The quick relief comes partly because the brain anticipates the effect of drinking, not because the body's fluid balance actually changes in that moment.[15] When predictions and signals match, everything feels natural and effortless. When they don't, we notice the mismatch—and that awareness helps the brain learn.

A *prediction error* occurs when the brain expects one thing, but the incoming signal suggests something different. The brain constantly anticipates what it thinks will happen, both around us and inside us. When signals don't match those expectations, it has to decide how to respond. It can update its expectations, learn from the new information, and slowly adjust. It might change behavior, acting to reduce discomfort or avoid what feels threatening. Or it can shift attention—amplifying a sensation or pushing it into the background. This process is a key way we learn and adapt.

Consider someone who was bitten by a dog as a child. Their brain might predict danger whenever they see a dog. Their heart races and their body prepares for a threat, even if the dog in front of them appears calm. If they gradually have safe experiences with friendly dogs, their brain may start to update its prediction. But if they avoid dogs altogether, the fear stays unchallenged and the expectation remains the same.

Prediction errors frequently appear in mental health struggles. Anxiety often involves the brain overestimating danger and interpreting normal bodily sensations as signs of threat. When someone struggles to identify emotions, emotional distress may show up mainly as physical symptoms—tightness in the chest, stomach pain, or fatigue—without a clear awareness of the underlying feeling.

These patterns help explain why interoception plays such a central role in both suffering and healing. When we learn to notice bodily signals with curiosity rather than immediate alarm, the brain (and our nervous system) has a better chance of updating its predictions and becoming more flexible. We'll revisit this in Chapter 6 when we explore how thinking patterns shape interoceptive experience.

## Space to Explore

Although research has come a long way, the science of interoception is still unfolding. Compared to other sensory systems, much is still unknown—and with every new discovery, more questions arise. This creates space for curiosity, growth, and ongoing exploration. Scientists are working to understand what these sensations mean, how they support well-being, and how they can become disrupted. As we've seen, interoception is a complex mind–body process with far-reaching effects. Continued research will deepen our understanding and offer new ways to support both physical and mental health.

# 3

# Interoception in Daily Life

In the previous chapter, we explored how various bodily systems send interoceptive messages and how these processes help maintain physical functioning. But our mental functions and understanding of our experiences in the world are also rooted in our bodies and in how we interact with our environment. Our bodies play a fundamental role in shaping our thoughts, perceptions, and emotions, and interoception is central to how we experience and regulate emotions. It enables us to notice emotional signals in the body and assess their intensity, which in turn helps us respond with the right tools to manage those emotions effectively. The way we interpret sensory signals affects everything from decision-making to how we react on a difficult day.

Interoception also plays a key role in shaping our sense of self. These internal signals serve as a physical anchor for self-identity, helping us understand who we are from within. This inward awareness is vital for emotional and social well-being. And just as interoception helps us connect with ourselves, it also supports our relationships with others—informing boundaries, empathy, and the reading of social cues. In this way, bodily sensations, emotions, thoughts, and relationships are not separate parts of life but interconnected experiences rooted in the body.

## Interoception and Emotional Experience

Interesting fact: People born blind still smile when they are happy, despite never having seen a happy facial expression. Researchers suggest that smiling is an innate and universal response to happiness.[1] This finding shows the connection between our physical bodies and our emotions—a connection we also see in how we describe feelings through bodily sensations. We get "butterflies in our stomachs" when we're anxious, or something that causes tension can be "a pain in the neck." A previous chapter introduced the idea that bodily sensations help form the basis for emotions through affective interoceptive messages. These internal signals blend physical sensations with emotional states, shaping our feelings and behaviors.

Interoceptive processes contribute to several distinct aspects of our emotional experience:

**Emotional awareness.** Interoception is how we notice the sensory signals coming from our bodies, forming the basis of emotional awareness and experience. For example, an increased heart rate and muscle tension are often associated with frustration or excitement. When people are more attuned to their bodily signals, they are more likely to notice and identify their emotions.

**Emotional differentiation.** Interoceptive awareness helps us not only identify but also differentiate what we're feeling. Many emotions generate similar physical sensations, and the differences can be subtle—a racing heart and tense muscles might indicate excitement or frustration. By tuning in to internal cues, we can use context and additional bodily signals to better understand our experiences.

**Emotional intensity.** Interoception also influences how strongly we feel our emotions. Some research suggests that individuals who are more sensitive to internal bodily signals, such as their heartbeat, may experience emotions more intensely, though this can depend on how those sensations are understood and responded to.[2]

**Emotional regulation.** When we can recognize our internal sensations—like rising anxiety or frustration—we're better able to regulate our emotions. Interoceptive awareness helps us notice shifts earlier, preventing them from escalating. Accurate identification makes it easier to choose helpful coping strategies; it's difficult to regulate what we cannot feel.

**Embodied emotions.** At its core, the word *embody* comes from Latin roots meaning "in the body." Here, embodiment refers to being fully present in and connected to our physical body. This connection is essential for understanding interoception and the mind–body relationship. Emotions aren't just mental states; they're rooted in bodily sensations.

## Interoception and Thinking

Interoception doesn't just help us manage bodily needs and emotions—it also plays a crucial role in rational thinking, learning, and decision-making. For example, if I'm dehydrated, I'll likely spend my last dollar on water rather than chips (no matter how much I might crave the chips). This simple choice reflects how bodily sensations inform our decisions. This concept challenges the traditional Western view of rational thought, expressed in René Descartes' "I think, therefore I am." The heart of Antonio Damasio's book *Descartes' Error* is that emotion is foundational to rational thinking and decision-making rather than separate from it, as Descartes implied.[3]

Damasio's research with brain-damaged patients, including the well-known case of Elliot, clearly illustrates this. After a brain tumor was removed, Elliot lost the ability to feel emotion. Although his intelligence and logical reasoning remained intact, his decision-making collapsed. He made choices that ruined his finances and relationships because he no longer had emotional signals to guide his judgment. He became stuck over trivial decisions—such as which pen to use or where to eat—while making major life choices that caused serious harm. Damasio argues that this case shows why logic alone is not enough: Emotions provide the sense of value, relevance, and urgency that help us choose wisely. Without them, even a highly rational mind can lose its way.

Damasio also proposes that damaging the brain regions that link emotion to reasoning leads to flawed judgment, even when rational abilities remain intact. Emotions and their connection to bodily states are not merely pleasant additions that enrich life; they are essential to the decision-making process that supports health, wellness, and strong relationships. This highlights yet another valuable aspect of interoception and its crucial role in our well-being.[4]

Neuroscientist Bud Craig takes this idea further in *How Do You Feel?*, where he asserts that our internal sensations play a key role in shaping behavior and guiding decisions[5]—like reaching for water instead of a soda when we're thirsty. He flips Descartes' famous line into "I feel, therefore I am," highlighting that we're not just thinkers but emotional beings whose lives are deeply influenced by interoceptive experience. Craig notes that people who are more attuned to their bodies—such as those who can sense their heartbeat more accurately—tend to function better both emotionally and cognitively. They notice subtle cues in their environment more quickly, make stronger decisions, stay more focused, and follow their gut instincts with confidence.[6]

## Interoception and the Sense of Self

Antonio Damasio's research adds to our understanding of how the sense of self develops. His work suggests that our sense of self is not abstract or purely intellectual; rather, it is deeply rooted in our bodily experiences of sensation and emotion.[7] Unsurprisingly, interoceptive awareness also plays a crucial role in our ability to say, "This is me," because it contributes to the physical, emotional, and cognitive facets of who we are. We might call this *embodied cognition*.

Neuroscience suggests that we experience ourselves in two complementary ways. One is the narrative self—the story we tell about who we are, shaped by memories, traits, and identity over time. The other is the experiential self, grounded in present-moment awareness of sensations, emotions, and bodily signals. Research on mindfulness indicates that these two forms of self-awareness rely on different brain networks. When attention shifts toward immediate experience—including bodily sensations—brain activity moves toward sensory and interoceptive regions such as the insula.[8] Together, these systems suggest that our sense of self arises both from the stories we tell about ourselves and from the body's signals in each moment.

Embodied cognition describes how our bodies and their interactions with the world shape emotional and cognitive processes. Our feelings, thoughts, and interpretations are grounded in sensory experience. In other words, our minds are not just "in our heads." Our thought processes and capacity for rational thinking are influenced by bodily experiences and sensations.

Let's look at four aspects of our sense of self—and it's no surprise that interoception is central to each one.

**Body and environment.** Signals like a racing heartbeat, the comfort of a chair beneath us, or the joy of a sunset remind us not only of our internal state but also that *This body is mine*. Self-awareness begins with that personal experience of *me*. Only I can feel my hunger, notice the pressure of my seat, or sense delight at something beautiful. Others can relate, but each of us experiences interoceptive cues from the inside out. Our sense of self—our thoughts, emotions, actions, and the feeling of *me*-ness—is rooted in this private, embodied awareness.

**Emotional experiences.** Our emotions are closely tied to bodily sensations, and together they shape our sense of who we are. Emotions reveal our needs, values, and preferences—they serve as an internal source of self-knowledge. Emotional awareness is also part of identity: My feelings arise within me; yours arise within you. Even when we share an event, we may interpret and feel it differently. Our emotional experiences are as unique as fingerprints—and they help define our sense of self as distinct from others.

**Sense of agency.** Agency is our ability to influence our lives through choices and actions. Every decision—from drinking a glass of water to pressing the snooze button—reflects an internal sense of control. Much of the time, this happens automatically; we go through our day on autopilot without conscious reflection. But when we become more aware of our ability to choose and act, our sense of self grows stronger. Noticing bodily cues and trusting them makes it easier to respond to our needs, regulate emotions before they escalate, and use coping strategies when stress rises. The more attuned we are to internal signals, the more empowered we are to take meaningful action.

**Self–other distinction.** Babies are not born with a clear sense of identity separate from their caregivers. This distinction begins to emerge around six months of age. Interoceptive and sensory feedback help infants learn that their body belongs to them. As children grow, that sense of separateness becomes more refined as they learn about their emotions, preferences, and cognitive processes. Interoception supports this self–other distinction by anchoring us in our own bodily signals while helping us recognize that someone else is separate from ourselves.

## Interoception and Social Connection

Another way interoception shows up in everyday life is through its impact on our relationships. It's no surprise that being aware of our internal bodily signals plays a role in forming and maintaining friendships. Think about the functions of interoception we've already covered—emotional awareness, self-regulation, and bodily awareness—and how essential they are when interacting with others. Our emotional awareness, grounded in bodily sensations, is key to connecting with people on a deeper level.

Interoception also supports our social understanding by helping us stay connected to ourselves. We need this sense of *me*-ness to recognize our thoughts and feelings as separate from someone else's. This self-awareness enables us to engage respectfully with others, respect their boundaries, and respond appropriately. Interoception enhances social intelligence by helping us read others' emotional cues more accurately, making us less likely to misinterpret their intentions or feelings. The interpersonal aspects of interoception are explored more fully in Chapter 19.

Learning to listen to the body also shapes how we experience emotions. Greater awareness of internal signals can clarify emotional experience, support regulation, and help us distinguish our own feelings from those around us. This self–other clarity allows for genuine empathy—feeling with another person without losing sight of our own perspective. Bud Craig put it well: People who are better at accurately detecting their heartbeat are better at recognizing their own emotions, and those who are better at recognizing their own feelings are better at recognizing the emotions of others.[9]

## Interoception and Mental Health

In recent years, scientists who study interoception have suggested that disrupted interoception is a common thread running through many mental health conditions, including depression, anxiety, PTSD, OCD, attention deficit hyperactivity disorder (ADHD), eating disorders, addiction disorders, self-harm, and suicidal ideation.[10] Some physical health issues influenced by psychological factors—such as asthma, chronic fatigue syndrome, and irritable bowel syndrome—are also linked to interoceptive dysfunction.

When we cannot accurately sense, interpret, or respond to our body's internal messages, our mental health suffers. Researchers note that understanding how the brain and body work together is becoming increasingly important for getting a complete picture of mental health.[11]

Mental health care has long focused on diagnosing people with specific "disorders" using systems like the *Diagnostic and Statistical Manual* (DSM). Most of us know the common labels—OCD, PTSD, depression, and so on. While these diagnoses can be helpful, many experts worry that the system is too quick to assign a label to someone without fully examining what is contributing to the problem.

That's why recent research is moving toward a *transdiagnostic approach*. Instead of viewing each diagnosis separately, this perspective looks for underlying processes that span many mental health conditions. One of those factors is interoception. Studies show that disruptions in the brain networks handling interoception are linked to a wide range of mental health struggles.[12] This suggests that many symptoms may stem from difficulties with interoceptive processes, not just from disorder-specific problems.

This perspective can be eye-opening. What appears to be multiple mental health issues might, in some cases, be different signs of impaired interoception. This helps explain why many conditions share similar features. Difficulties in sensing the body make emotional regulation more challenging—a common factor in PTSD, depression, anxiety, and substance use. Changes in self-perception, another key sign of disrupted interoception, are often seen in complex PTSD, body dysmorphia, and dissociative disorders.

Interoceptive difficulties also tend to add up. Struggles in one area—such as noticing bodily cues—can spill over into others, including emotion regulation. Difficulty managing emotions then affects relationships. When we're disconnected from our bodies and their signals, it creates a ripple effect that touches nearly every aspect of life. This is not a one-way process. Interoceptive challenges can influence emotions, emotions can disrupt relationships, relationship stress can impact mental health, and mental health struggles can further dysregulate the body. Each part of our lives affects the others, creating a loop—and interoceptive processes are a common thread running through it.

In my work as a therapist, I've seen how essential it is to include the body in therapy. It's not just helpful, it's necessary for real healing. Even before I learned the term *interoception*, I noticed how challenging it was for some clients to connect with their bodies. Some couldn't track what they were feeling, others felt overwhelmed by something as simple as noticing their breath, and some fixated on bodily sensations. Long before I began researching interoception, I was already witnessing these struggles in my clients. To me, this affirms the wisdom of traditional mind–body practices—reminding us that emotional and mental health live in the body, even before research gave us the language for it.

## How Interoceptive Disturbances Show Up

Although the main focus of Part 3 is the link between interoception and mental health, it's helpful to first examine the different ways interoceptive disruptions can develop. These disruptions can affect our physical, emotional, cognitive, mental, and relational well-being. As you read, you'll see that difficulties occur along a spectrum and can appear at both ends of human experience.

The story of Goldilocks provides a helpful metaphor. She wasn't looking for extremes—too hot or too cold—but for the balance of "just right." Interoception functions similarly. When it's working well, it helps us care for our bodies, regulate emotions, think clearly, and build healthy relationships. However, many people don't experience this balance. Some notice too few internal signals, while others feel overwhelmed by them. Some avoid bodily cues altogether, while others become excessively focused on them. Like Goldilocks, the goal is often to find a middle ground—a sense of "just right" inside ourselves.

## *Bodily Needs: Pushing Through or a Blank Page*

Interoceptive signals allow us to sense and respond to our body's needs, which is vital for physical and mental well-being. But for individuals who struggle in other areas of physical or emotional regulation, two extremes often emerge in how they interpret these signals.

Some may feel bodily signals but continue to push through them, consciously or unconsciously. They may ignore their need for food or sleep under deadline pressure. They may override those signals to keep binge-watching a show or playing a game. Pushing through pain, illness, and exhaustion is common among those who disregard their interoceptive messages—a pattern that increases the risk of burnout, mood changes, chronic health concerns, and difficulties with emotional regulation.

*Catherine is a perfectionist at work as a nurse and at home, where she cares for her three children. Her children are involved in many activities. She hosts most family holidays and never misses anyone's birthday. Catherine often pushes through hunger, fatigue, and pain to work an extra shift for a colleague, plan a family activity, or host a gathering.*

In contrast, some people have a very limited connection to their interoceptive cues—their bodies are experienced as "blank pages," with diminished sensory input. They often have difficulty noticing the signals their bodies send: They may not feel hunger or thirst cues or readily recognize the need to use the bathroom. They may be unaware of pain or illness, not realizing there is a problem until symptoms become severe. Some of these experiences are common among individuals who are neurodivergent.

*Roland, an accountant, has very little awareness of bodily sensations. When asked what he notices happening in his body, he usually responds, "Nothing." Recently, Roland was diagnosed with advanced symptoms of acid reflux. The only symptom he noticed was increased coughing. Given the damage to his stomach and esophagus, Roland's doctor was surprised that he did not seek help earlier.*

## *Experiencing Emotions: Coldhearted or Hot-Tempered*

Interoception influences how well we can recognize our feelings, how strongly we experience them, and how effectively we can use tools to manage them. When mental health challenges are present, it's common to see people skew toward the extremes rather than having a more balanced emotional experience.

Some individuals are disconnected from their emotions because they struggle to connect their feelings with the physical sensations they experience. To others, this can make them seem cold, emotionless, or numb. They may have difficulty recognizing when they're feeling something or may display a limited range of emotions. This can lead to confusion or make it hard for them to put their emotions into words. They may even deny feeling anything at all—like the person who insists, "I'm not angry," even though their body language and tone make it obvious to everyone else.

*Roland isn't just disconnected from bodily sensations; he's disconnected from emotions. He describes his life in concrete terms—work, routines, and tasks—but is unable to articulate feelings. He has difficulty identifying and expressing emotions and tends to devalue emotional experience, both for himself and his family. He approaches life issues and decisions from a cognitive perspective, emphasizing facts over subjective or emotional perspectives.*

On the other end of the spectrum are those who are more emotionally sensitive or reactive. They may feel things very deeply, very quickly, and for longer than others. Even small triggers can set off intense reactions, and calming down may take some time. They may be easily angered and respond impulsively or hurtfully to others. For these individuals, the challenge isn't a lack of feeling; it's feeling something so intensely that managing emotional responses becomes difficult.

*Jason has been let go from several construction crews due to aggressive outbursts and unsafe behavior. Along with the assault charge against him and employment instability, he is known to be confrontational when provoked. Because Jason has little awareness of what is happening in his body, he blames others for his outbursts. He doesn't realize that his frustration has been building long before a blowup.*

## *Rational Thinking: Reckless Choices or Analysis Paralysis*

Bodily sensations and experiences influence our thinking and decision-making skills. Yet those with disrupted interoception often miss or doubt the internal cues that help shape rational thought. For example, some people cannot use bodily sensations to guide their decisions. They tend to make impulsive or reckless choices, especially if their body is under stress that their brain isn't registering. In healthy decision-making, our bodies can offer warning signals or confirm that a choice is sound. A racing heart or muscle tension can signal a stressful situation. Without these interoceptive cues, individuals are more likely to act impulsively or make poor judgments.

*It shouldn't be surprising that Jason struggles with impulsivity and reckless choices. In addition to his aggressive behavior at work and in his personal life, he also takes unnecessary risks while driving. Since Jason has a poor connection to his bodily sensations, he struggles to recognize early warning signs of growing tension or stress. What appears to be a reckless choice is most often emotional reactivity.*

The opposite problem occurs for those who tend to overthink. *Analysis paralysis* is a state of overthinking in which someone spends too long deliberating over a situation or problem because no option feels *right.* This often happens to people who struggle to connect with their emotional and physical sensations. Decision-making can also become difficult for individuals who struggle to prioritize options and determine what matters most. They may even mistrust their gut feelings, making the process exhausting.

*Lauren, a preschool teacher, can read others like an open book but struggles to understand herself. She's great at listening to others but isn't always aware of the messages her body sends. Lauren often seeks guidance from others for personal decisions or spends excessive time online researching every option. She gets caught in analysis paralysis, delays making decisions, and is plagued by endless what-ifs.*

## *Sense of Self: People-Pleasing and Egomania*

Ideally, interoceptive cues provide an accurate sense of self-awareness. They contribute to our experience of agency and shape how we perceive ourselves in relation to others. When our sense of self is rooted in our physical experiences and sensations, we gain a deeper understanding of who we are. However, when someone has difficulty interpreting interoceptive signals, they may develop an overly inflated view of themselves—or an unrealistically low opinion of their needs and self-worth.

People pleasers often sacrifice themselves to meet others' needs. Their challenges with interoception make it harder for them to sense, interpret, or act upon their own needs. Their sense of self is shaped more by external cues, such as the desire for validation or the fear of disapproval, than by their own wants. Those with a diminished connection to themselves may also ignore their own signals of stress or fatigue, continuing to say *yes* to others.

Recognizing and maintaining personal boundaries become harder when people are disconnected from their physical and emotional cues.

> *Catherine works hard to meet everyone's needs—except her own. She automatically says yes whenever someone asks for something. No matter what is requested, she fulfills it. Catherine's self-worth is tied to how much she can give. She rarely considers her own physical or emotional needs. Even when she's exhausted, the thought of disappointing someone feels unbearable.*

Challenges with interoception and reduced emotional awareness can also fuel an inflated ego. Interoceptive difficulties may prevent someone from feeling discomfort when they've been overconfident. They might struggle to interpret social cues that offer feedback on how others perceive them. And when a person can't connect to bodily sensations, they're more likely to rely on self-perceptions often shaped by distorted thoughts.

> *At first glance, Ava appears self-assured. But a closer look reveals a different picture. She is boastful and overconfident yet craves constant admiration. She dismisses negative comments as jealousy. She has very few female friends because other young women see her as self-centered. Beneath her confident exterior, her self-worth is entirely dependent on the attention she gets from others.*

## *Interpersonal Relationships: Overempathy and Narcissism*

Interoceptive challenges can deeply affect our relationships. Because emotional awareness and emotional regulation are central aspects of interoception, difficulties sensing internal cues often influence how we connect with others. Interoception helps us maintain a healthy sense of self—staying attuned to our own emotions while remaining open to others. When this balance is disrupted, relationships may become strained. For example, high empathy and narcissistic tendencies are opposite relational patterns that are partly shaped by interoceptive awareness.

People with narcissistic traits often have difficulty recognizing others' emotions because they are less attuned to their own, except for those that boost their self-image. This disconnect from internal signals can lead to an unstable or inflated sense of self that depends heavily on admiration or status, making it harder to build secure and meaningful relationships.

> *Ava often appears self-absorbed, making others unsure whether she truly cares about anyone else. Her parents are frustrated because she*

*uses their home as her personal studio, and when they set boundaries, she responds with tears, anger, and accusations that they do not support her dreams. She also uses her social media profile to attract men who are willing to buy the expensive jewelry and clothing she features in her posts.*

While empathy is essential for healthy relationships, some people struggle with experiencing "too much" empathy. These individuals excel at recognizing interoceptive cues related to emotions, both their own and those of others; after all, interoception helps us feel empathy and understand others' feelings. But excessive empathy can blur the lines between our experiences and those of others. This can lead to feeling overwhelmed by another person's emotions or drained by the intensity of emotionally charged situations.

*In many ways, Lauren is well-suited to her work with children because she is highly sensitive to others' emotional needs. This makes her a caring teacher and friend—until the lines blur between herself and others. She often feels she absorbs the anxiety or sadness of those around her, which leaves her emotionally and physically depleted by the end of the day.*

We've only begun to explore the many ways impaired interoception can impact well-being. The next chapter examines how interoception is measured in research and clinical settings and introduces the Multidimensional Assessment of Interoceptive Awareness (MAIA), which helps us understand interoception as a set of skills we can strengthen over time.

# 4

# How Interoception Is Measured

With a clearer understanding of both the biology and application of interoception, we can now explore how to study it and how individuals or clinicians can develop a more personalized understanding of interoceptive awareness. This foundation also helps us see how interoceptive processes may change or develop in time.

Science depends on reliable measurement to build knowledge, but studying interoception makes that especially tricky. Interoception involves private, subjective sensations, which are difficult to measure and quantify. People's interoceptive abilities also vary widely, so there's no clear baseline for what counts as "normal." Still, researchers recognize the importance of studying it, even if the science is a bit messy. Take the heartbeat perception test: It's one of the most common ways to measure interoception, yet about 40 percent of people can't consciously feel their heartbeat.[1] So if you can't either, you're not alone.

The terminology itself can add to the confusion. Definitions of interoceptive constructs are often vague and difficult to operationalize. Different researchers may use the same terms in different ways. For example, *interoceptive sensitivity* might refer to accurately counting heartbeats in one study, while in another it could mean being generally aware of internal sensations. This lack of consistency makes the field challenging to study—but also exciting, as new methods and clearer definitions continue to emerge.

## Challenges with Measuring Interoception

Researchers face several challenges when measuring interoceptive awareness: differences across body systems, the complexity of interoception itself, questions of accuracy, and the balance between objective and subjective methods.

**Different body systems are sensed differently.** As we saw in Chapter 2, interoceptive signals originate from many places, but the heart and stomach are the most commonly studied. The heartbeat perception test measures an individual's ability to sense their own heartbeat, while the water load test assesses cues of stomach fullness. Interestingly, being good at one doesn't guarantee being good at the other.[2] Many people cannot feel their heartbeat at all. This tells us that our ability to sense what's happening inside our bodies isn't uniform—it varies widely across systems and from person to person.

**Interoception involves complex skills.** Interoception is complex. It's not just about noticing bodily signals—it's also about interpreting them accurately and trusting what they mean. Rather than a single ability, interoception is better understood as a set of related skills. Because these skills differ from one another, measuring interoception isn't straightforward. It can even be challenging to determine which aspects to test, since different traits and abilities contribute to the overall picture.

**Accuracy is difficult to assess.** Tests like heartbeat counting can be unreliable and often impractical. People vary greatly in their abilities, and some may even guess their heart rate, reducing accuracy. Similar issues arise with gastrointestinal and respiratory tests. In the GI domain, methods such as inflating a small balloon in the stomach or using drink-based fullness tests can be invasive, uncomfortable, and hard to standardize. In the respiratory domain, tasks that require breathing through a tube to detect increased resistance or changes in carbon dioxide ($CO_2$) can feel unpleasant and stressful. These tests also lack precision and tend to yield unreliable results.[3]

**Objective and subjective measures each have limits.** Researchers use both objective and subjective measures. Objective methods, such as heartbeat detection tasks or tests of sensitivity to rising $CO_2$ levels, are often impractical and may lack precision. Subjective measures rely on self-reports about how confident people feel in noticing and trusting their body's signals, but these have their own limitations. For example, they cannot be validated against an objective gold standard, because no such standard exists for many aspects of interoceptive awareness. Additionally, questionnaires carry familiar challenges, including response bias, shifting emotional states, and the tendency to answer in ways that present oneself positively rather than with complete honesty.[4] Both approaches offer value, yet neither is perfect.

## Making Sense of the Science of Interoception

Science is constantly evolving, and the study of interoception is advancing quickly. What we understand now will continue to shift as researchers develop new ways to explore this inner sense. Measuring interoception is particularly difficult because no single test is fully reliable, valid, and practical. As a result, scientists will continue experimenting with new approaches.

Olivier Desmedt and colleagues have reviewed many of these methods and reached an interesting conclusion: Interoceptive accuracy may not be the most important focus.[5] What matters more is whether people can notice their bodily signals, make sense of them, and trust what they mean. Sarah Garfinkel, an interoception pioneer who helped develop the heartbeat perception test, and her colleague Chatrin Suksasilp now emphasize the value of examining expectations or beliefs about bodily cues rather than accuracy alone. They note that self-reported beliefs reveal new ways to understand mental health challenges like anxiety and depression.[6]

This shift in thinking echoes the words of William Bruce Cameron: "Not everything that counts can be counted, and not everything that can be counted counts."[7] In other words, some of the most important aspects of interoception—such as how we interpret and respond to our inner signals—may not fit neatly into standard measures, yet they remain vital for understanding health and well-being.

As a therapist, I'm especially interested in my clients' subjective interoceptive experiences: how they perceive bodily sensations and whether they can listen to and trust what their bodies are telling them. It makes sense to focus on these personal experiences and beliefs rather than solely on how accurate someone is at noticing cues. Like Goldilocks searching for *just right*, interoception is about balance. Some people struggle to notice signals, others ignore or push past them, and still others feel overwhelmed by them. How people interpret and respond to their body's messages has been a central part of my work with clients.

## A Helpful Way to Assess Interoception

Understanding individual differences in interoceptive experiences is key to linking altered interoception with mental health concerns. How a person perceives and interprets their bodily sensations offers valuable insights into this sensory system and can highlight specific challenges they may face. One of the most widely used tools for this purpose is the Multidimensional

Assessment of Interoceptive Awareness (MAIA), first developed by Wolf Mehling and his research team in 2012 and later updated in 2018 (MAIA-2).[8]

The MAIA-2 is a self-report questionnaire with thirty-seven statements covering eight different aspects, or domains, of interoceptive awareness. Participants rate each statement on a scale from *never* to *always*. Examples include "I notice when I am uncomfortable in my body" and "I try to ignore pain." These items reveal how people perceive, respond to, and regulate their bodily sensations. Importantly, the MAIA-2 assesses both adaptive aspects of interoception—such as tuning in to and trusting sensations—and less helpful patterns, such as ignoring or feeling overwhelmed by them.

The questionnaire's thirty-seven statements map onto eight areas of interoceptive awareness: noticing, not-distracting, not-worrying, attention regulation, emotional awareness, self-regulation, body listening, and trusting. As you read through the descriptions of these domains—presented in the following pages alongside case studies—you may begin to recognize your own interoceptive tendencies. The case studies illustrate different patterns of altered interoception, while an additional example of an individual with adaptive interoceptive skills shows how these patterns vary from person to person. Throughout the book, we will continue to revisit the MAIA and these clients to explore how interoception is shaped by stress, trauma, anxiety, depression, and other mental and emotional health challenges.

If you are interested in taking the MAIA-2 yourself, you can do so by visiting www.carriedejong.com/maia.

### 1. Noticing: Awareness of Physical Sensations

***Example:*** *When I am tense, I notice where the tension is located in my body.*

Noticing interoceptive cues means tuning in to signals from the body—breathing, warmth, tension, a full bladder, digestion, and other sensations. These cues can be pleasant, unpleasant, or neutral, and paying attention to them offers insight into our physical state, emotions, and stress responses. The key is to notice without judgment or trying to change anything, simply observing what's happening.

This skill forms the foundation of interoceptive awareness. When we tune in, we better understand our bodies and emotions, which helps us care for ourselves, think more clearly, and connect more deeply with others. Someone skilled at noticing bodily sensations might use those cues to guide their everyday choices:

*John gets home after a long, stressful day at work. He had planned to go for a run, but he notices he's exhausted and hungry. He's also aware that he's still irritated from a challenging conversation with a colleague.*

People vary widely in how they notice their sensations.

*Roland, Ava, and Jason are all quite disconnected from their physical sensations: Roland isn't aware of emotional cues and doesn't notice the discomfort of acid reflux. Jason can't detect early warning signs of tension or agitation. Ava disregards her feelings of hunger.*

*Catherine registers cues like fatigue and pain but typically dismisses them so she can keep pushing herself.*

*David notices sensations, but his ability to do so is muted. His awareness is also filtered through his chronic fatigue and lethargy.*

*Lauren and Hailey both score higher in this area: Lauren tends to be highly attuned to her sensations, especially those linked to others' emotions, which she feels keenly. Hailey notices nearly every internal shift in sensation and constantly monitors her body.*

## 2. Not-Distracting: Tendency Not to Ignore or Distract from Uncomfortable Sensations

***Example:*** *I push feelings of discomfort away by focusing on something else.*

Not distracting from interoceptive sensations means noticing bodily cues without ignoring or avoiding them, even when they're uncomfortable. Instead of numbing or pushing past pain through habits like emotional eating, substance use, or constant busyness, this skill encourages openness and acceptance. While distraction may bring short-term relief, it often makes it more difficult to meet physical and emotional needs.

Higher scores in this area reflect greater acceptance of unpleasant sensations—not because we enjoy them, but because we can tolerate them. This capacity is seen as a positive trait, linked to stronger self-awareness and better management of physical and emotional challenges. Lower scores suggest a tendency to suppress or avoid discomfort, which can increase stress and delay care. The ability to stay with discomfort reflects a healthier, more balanced relationship with the body.

*Sometimes John rehashes tough conversations after work and feels frustrated about how he handled them. Other nights, he might go for a run to clear his mind, but tonight he's too tired. Part of him wants to tune out and watch something mindless to escape the discomfort. Instead, he decides to cook an easy meal to take care of himself.*

Across the following case studies, all clients score low in this area, indicating that they typically distract themselves from, ignore, or suppress their bodily sensations.

*Roland does not notice uncomfortable sensations in the first place, so he has little need to distract from them. He suppresses discomfort rather than consciously avoiding it.*

*Catherine is a people pleaser who often ignores bodily discomfort or pushes through fatigue and hunger to meet expectations and get things done. When she needs a break, she distracts herself with alcohol.*

*Ava and Jason both distract from bodily sensations: Ava distracts by focusing on her appearance, seeking attention, or scrolling on her phone when she feels emotional or physical discomfort. Jason distracts or numbs himself with cannabis or alcohol.*

*Lauren and Hailey have a low tolerance for discomfort and react immediately to even mild unpleasant sensations.*

*David habitually escapes discomfort rather than attending to it, often through food or time on his phone.*

### 3. Not-Worrying: Tendency Not to Worry About Unpleasant Sensations or Respond with Distress

***Example:*** *I start to worry that something is wrong if I feel any discomfort.*

This aspect of interoceptive awareness reflects how much we worry about bodily sensations. Not worrying means staying reasonably calm with discomfort—such as pain or tension—rather than spiraling into anxious thoughts. People who score higher here can notice unpleasant sensations and use healthy coping strategies without becoming overwhelmed.

*When John pauses and notices his fatigue, a familiar thought pops up:* If I skip my run, I'm losing my discipline. *That worry could easily push him to run anyway. Instead, he acknowledges the thought and then checks in with his body to see what it truly needs. By letting go of the worry about missing one workout, John allows his body—rather than his fears—to guide his decisions.*

Those who worry more often get caught in overthinking, catastrophic thinking, and distress, which, ironically, increase their discomfort. It becomes a vicious cycle. A healthier approach is to notice the body's cues with curiosity instead of fear, building a stronger and more balanced mind–body connection.

*Roland and Jason both score in the middle: Roland is unconcerned about symptoms like acid reflux, but his lack of worry stems from detachment and denial rather than healthy coping. Jason suppresses and minimizes his emotional tension and believes he is "fine"—until he eventually explodes.*

*Catherine also scores in the mid-range. She generally doesn't worry about her bodily sensations, but she interprets pain or fatigue as signs of weakness. This increases her self-criticism and pushes her to keep going rather than rest.*

*Ava worries about gaining weight and feeling bloated, which greatly upsets her.*

*Lauren and Hailey have low scores. Both tend to worry about and catastrophize their bodily sensations, often feeling anxiety about physical symptoms, which adds to their emotional distress.*

*David also scores low. He interprets tension or fatigue through a negative lens and assumes they reflect personal failure.*

## 4. Attention Regulation: Ability to Regulate Attention to Bodily Sensations

***Example:*** *I can return awareness to my body if I am distracted.*

This capacity involves mindfully engaging with bodily sensations, such as noticing your heartbeat, breath, or muscle tension, and bringing your attention back when your mind wanders. The goal is finding balance: staying aware without becoming disconnected or overwhelmed.

Attentional regulation helps us distinguish between anxiety, excitement, or even indigestion, and recognize whether we're reacting to hunger or frustration. People who score lower in this area may struggle to stay connected to their bodily cues and may become easily distracted. The ability to *stay with* sensations supports self-care, deepens self-understanding, and strengthens emotional regulation.

*John's work has stressful and demanding aspects. He can get caught in the flurry of meetings and deadlines and forget to eat, breathe, or take a posture break. He is learning to pause and refocus on what his body needs, even when he is absorbed in external demands.*

None of our examples score well in this area:

*Roland has the least capacity to focus inward. His attention is directed almost entirely toward tasks, routines, and his thoughts.*

*Catherine struggles to notice her internal state until she feels exhausted or overwhelmed.*

*Ava directs nearly all of her attention outward—to cameras, mirrors, and her audience's reactions.*

*Jason also has difficulty focusing inward and has limited awareness of his emotional or bodily states.*

*Lauren can pay some attention to her internal cues, but she tends to focus on the negative ones, especially when she is tired or in pain.*

*Hailey can't attend to her bodily sensations without experiencing fear and anxiety.*

## 5. Emotional Awareness: Ability to Recognize the Connection Between Bodily Sensations and Emotions

***Example:*** *I notice how my body changes when I feel happy or joyful.*

Emotional awareness is the ability to recognize how emotions manifest in the body. How do we notice tension when stressed, a racing heart when scared, or butterflies when excited? It's more than labeling feelings; it's experiencing emotions through the sensations our bodies produce.

When we're tuned in, it becomes easier to distinguish subtle emotions—is it anger or fear, excitement or anxiety? This awareness not only deepens self-understanding but also helps us regulate emotions more skillfully. Those who struggle to link body sensations with feelings often find it harder to cope in healthy ways. Greater emotional awareness, on the other hand, builds resilience, strengthens connection, and promotes a more balanced emotional life.

*If an email frustrates him, John notices the warm flush in his face and the tension in his hands. Instead of firing off a quick, reactive response, he labels the emotion—*I'm annoyed*—and waits until his body settles before replying.*

The results for emotional awareness vary and reveal some interesting nuances:

*Roland's ability to recognize and understand his emotions is severely limited. He cannot link bodily cues with feelings and struggles to name or describe what he's experiencing.*

*Catherine scores in the mid-range. Although she can recognize her emotions, she filters them through her self-judgment and believes she "shouldn't" feel tired or annoyed.*

*Ava experiences her emotions intensely, but her low interoceptive awareness makes it harder to interpret what those sensations mean. She struggles to use those sensations to understand herself or to regulate her responses when upset.*

*Jason can't connect sensations (such as a racing heart or tight chest) with feelings like frustration or rising anger. Instead, his emotions tend to be expressed behaviorally.*

*Lauren scores very high in this area. As someone who identifies as an empath, she is highly attuned to the connection between emotions and bodily sensations.*

*Hailey has some emotional awareness but finds it difficult to distinguish between physical sensations of anxiety and signs of actual medical illness.*

*David is unable to read bodily sensations as emotional cues. Instead, he disconnects and numbs feelings of grief, sadness, or stress.*

## 6. Self-Regulation: Ability to Regulate Distress Through Attention to Bodily Sensations

***Example:*** *I can use my breath to reduce tension.*

Self-regulation involves matching bodily sensations with appropriate emotional and behavioral responses. How effectively can we notice cues like tension or a racing heart and use them to guide our actions? Do we manage frustration in healthy ways, such as taking a break or slowing our breathing to calm ourselves when stressed?

People who score higher in this area manage emotions more effectively, notice early warning signs, and respond thoughtfully rather than reacting impulsively. They use tools like deep breathing or muscle relaxation to stay grounded. Building interoceptive self-regulation strengthens resilience and supports better mental health.

*Although giving presentations is a routine part of John's work, he still finds them stressful. When he feels tension in his stomach and energy in his chest, he uses a calming breath tool to settle his nervous system and prepare himself mentally.*

You may have guessed that all the individuals in these case studies have lower scores in this area:

*Roland has the weakest connection to his sensations. As a result, he has almost no ability to regulate his emotions or behaviors in healthy ways. It's impossible to regulate something that isn't being felt.*

*Catherine has very few healthy tools for self-regulation. She tends to rely on alcohol to manage her internal discomfort.*

*Ava lacks strategies to soothe distress. Instead, she seeks external validation or distracts herself with exercise. Her dependence on external regulation leads to further emotional instability.*

*Jason cannot recognize his growing frustration, which prevents him from using tools such as grounding, breathing, or taking a break to calm his stress response. As a result, his behavior becomes reactive and his anger goes unchecked.*

*Lauren can practice healthy self-care at times, but when she is overwhelmed by pain or by others' emotions, she struggles to find calm.*

*Hailey has very few skills to soothe herself when she begins to experience anxiety.*

*David's depression diminishes his motivation and energy, which makes it difficult for him to engage in self-care.*

## *7. Body Listening: Ability to Actively Listen to the Body for Insight or Guidance*

***Example:*** *I listen for information from my body about my emotional state.*
Body listening means tuning in to our inner signals and using them to guide choices and self-care. It's about listening to our "gut sense." This involves not just noticing sensations but also interpreting them—resting when we're tired, exploring our emotions, or paying attention to subtle cues.

People who listen to their bodies treat these signals as valuable information, which builds self-awareness and enables healthier responses to stress, emotions, and physical needs. Those who struggle with this skill often miss important signs about their well-being. Developing body listening strengthens our connection to ourselves and supports overall health.

*When John notices cues of fatigue, hunger, and irritation, he chooses to stretch after eating and then take a short walk instead of ignoring what his body is telling him.*

None of the individuals in these case studies listen to their bodies for insight or guidance:

*Roland and Jason both have significantly diminished abilities to listen to their bodies: Roland rarely notices sensation cues that could offer clues about his emotions or physical health. Jason is similarly disconnected from his internal signals.*

*Catherine seldom listens to her body for guidance. She pushes through internal cues to meet her high standards, basing her decisions on "shoulds" and others' expectations rather than her own needs.*

*Ava treats her body as something to display rather than as a source of guidance. She ignores signals of fatigue, hunger, or stress in pursuit of the validation she craves.*

*Lauren and Hailey also do poorly in this area. Both tend to misinterpret what their sensations are trying to communicate. Instead of viewing interoceptive cues as helpful information, they see them as sources of fear and anxiety.*

## 8. Trusting: Experience of One's Body as Safe and Trustworthy

***Example:*** *I am at home in my body.*

Trusting bodily sensations means believing that our bodies are safe and reliable sources of information. It reflects an inner sense of security, recognizing our bodily cues as accurate and trustworthy. It enables us to approach discomfort with curiosity and care rather than fear or avoidance. When we feel safe in our bodies, it becomes easier to listen to the signals they send and use them to guide self-care.

When body trust is low, people often feel disconnected and mistrustful of their sensations, which makes healthy choices more difficult. Building this trust is essential for resilience, healing, and a stronger sense of self.

*When John notices he's feeling tired after a busy morning at work, he doesn't question whether he's "letting his team down." He trusts the sensation as valid information and adjusts by taking a brief walk, grabbing a snack, or slowing his pace at work.*

It won't be surprising that everyone in these case studies scores low on their ability to trust the sensations their bodies produce:

*Roland deeply mistrusts his body signals, often viewing them as irrelevant or misleading. He disregards both medical advice and his wife's concerns.*

*Catherine pushes against her body rather than trusting it. Because her self-worth depends on performance, she finds it difficult to see her body's signals as valid or helpful.*

*Ava's impulse to "fix" or distract from sensations shows little trust in her body and reflects a belief that her internal cues are problems to eliminate rather than information to consider.*

*Jason considers his bodily signals unreliable. Since he can't recognize or monitor his rising frustration, he ignores his physical cues and blames others for his aggression.*

*Lauren doesn't trust her bodily signals or use them for guidance. Although she's very aware of her sensations, she often misinterprets them and relies heavily on external input, such as online searches and others' opinions, especially when something affects her personally.*

*Hailey sees her body as fragile and vulnerable to disease, which makes it difficult for her to trust the sensations she experiences.*

* * *

People can struggle with interoceptive awareness in different ways. Although measuring interoception precisely is difficult, tools like the MAIA-2 provide a richer picture of an individual's subjective experience of this sensory "superpower." For therapists and mental health professionals, it serves as a valuable guide for identifying challenges and shaping targeted interventions. For people interested in strengthening their mind–body connection, it offers a roadmap for understanding both interoceptive challenges and existing resources. We'll dig deeper into this in the chapters ahead.

# Part Two

# WHAT SHAPES OUR INTEROCEPTIVE EXPERIENCES

# 5

# Miscommunication Between Body and Brain

Who hasn't experienced the frustrations of navigating video calls and the potential for glitches that disrupt the quality of communication? Someone can't get their video feed to turn on. Another forgets to mute during a conference call, and suddenly we're eavesdropping on their conversation with the dog groomer. A device isn't charged, so it dies mid-call. Video communications can add a whole new layer of challenge to a conversation.

Miscommunication happens in writing, too. Think about how punctuation changes the meaning of this sentence: "I like cooking my family and my pets" sounds rather ominous. Add a few commas, and the meaning shifts entirely. Instead of a confession by a psychopath, it becomes a statement of affection: "I like cooking, my family, and my pets." This is a good reminder of the power of the humble comma.

We all understand communication challenges, whether it's poor cell service or a misunderstood text message. The challenges are similar in interoceptive processes. Interoception is a constant two-way exchange between the body and the brain, and just like technology, that conversation can get interrupted. Signals may not come through clearly, they may be misunderstood, or they may be missed altogether.

Understanding how our interoceptive experiences are shaped and what can disrupt them is crucial. In Part 2 of this book, we examine these influences in detail. Illness, thought patterns, life events, and relationships all affect how we sense and interpret our inner world. In the rest of this chapter, we'll focus on *bottom-up* challenges, in which issues in the body—such as illness, injury, gut health, or certain behaviors—disrupt messages sent to the brain. The next chapter turns to *top-down* challenges, showing how thoughts and beliefs can interfere with a healthy body–brain dialogue. Later chapters explore how early attachment patterns, stress, and trauma further shape how interoception works.

## Hypersensitivity and Hyposensitivity

Think back to Goldilocks and her search for *just right*. Interoception can work the same way. For some people, the body's signals are too loud—like being at a concert where the volume is overwhelming. For others, the signals are too faint, like someone speaking softly in a noisy room. As a result, they miss much of the message. And then there's the middle ground: the just-right zone, where signals come through clearly enough to notice but not so strongly that they drown everything else out. Researchers and clinicians often refer to these extremes as *hypersensitivity* (over) and *hyposensitivity* (under). The sweet spot in between helps us recognize and respond to our body's cues in a more balanced, healthy way.

Let's apply this lens to the individuals we met in previous chapters.

*Roland misses most of the messages his body sends, leaving him without valuable cues that could guide his decisions and support his health. For him, the volume of bodily communication is so low that it's barely perceptible.*

*Jason is more complex, showing a mix of both extremes. He feels emotions like anger so intensely that they erupt impulsively. At the same time, he struggles to regulate those reactions—suggesting that some interoceptive channels are too loud, while others are muted.*

*Lauren is highly aware of her sensations and often perceives them too intensely. Her sensitivity extends to others as well: She picks up on others' emotional cues so strongly that they become overwhelming rather than helpful.*

*Hailey notices every shift in her body and interprets each sensation as an alarm. For her, heightened awareness fuels anxiety, creating a loop in which noticing leads directly to increased distress.*

## How Interoceptive Sensitivity Impacts Health and Mental Health

Research provides valuable insight into how interoceptive sensitivity affects physical and mental health, showing that oversensitivity to body signals can increase vulnerability to anxiety and panic.[1] For instance, someone with panic disorder might notice minor changes—like a racing heart or shallow breathing—that can escalate into worry about what those sensations mean.

*The more attention Hailey gives to her bodily sensations, the more anxious she becomes. This creates a vicious cycle: certain sensations trigger fear, the fear amplifies the sensations, and the intensified sensations fuel her health anxiety even further.*

Interoceptive processes and hypersensitivity also play a significant role in chronic pain.[2] In conditions like fibromyalgia, irritable bowel syndrome (IBS), and chronic migraine, individuals often exhibit heightened awareness of internal sensations, especially those related to pain. Unfortunately, hypersensitivity can worsen symptoms. The pain signals can get so intense that they drown out all other sensations.

*When caregiving overwhelms Lauren, it triggers fatigue and IBS. In turn, the pain worsens her emotional distress, creating a harmful feedback loop. Her increased emotional sensitivity leaves her feeling overwhelmed, which then amplifies her pain and exhaustion, leading to even more stress and discomfort.*

At the other end are people whose body signals come through too faintly. This blunted sensitivity, or hyposensitivity, is common in conditions like depression.[3] Here, important bodily cues get missed or misunderstood, making it harder to meet physical and emotional needs. Later chapters will explore how these patterns affect both mental and physical health.

*Roland's sensitivity to bodily cues is so low that he misses almost all emotional experiences. He can't recognize the physical signals alerting him that his acid reflux is damaging his esophagus. He also shows clear signs of chronic stress but doesn't realize how much it affects him.*

Interestingly, a significant portion of recent interoceptive research has focused on neurodiversity. It is common for autistic people to be highly sensitive to external sensory experiences. Kelly Mahler, an occupational therapist, has developed extensive resources linking interoceptive deficits to challenges faced by autistic individuals. She contributed to an article highlighting how bodily cues are often unnoticed or misunderstood in autistic children.[4] Too much visual or auditory stimulation can be overwhelming, and a similar pattern often appears in their responses to interoceptive sensations. Some experience greater distress from uncomfortable bodily cues, while others show the opposite pattern: a high tolerance for pain and difficulty recognizing internal signals like hunger or thirst.[5]

With ADHD, a slightly different pattern emerges. Research indicates that interoceptive sensitivity is often decreased.[6] People may be less aware of their bodily signals, leading to missed signs of fatigue and difficulty recognizing when it's time to rest. This reduced sensitivity is also connected to impulsivity and risk-taking. When the body's warning cues are less apparent, it becomes easier to overlook danger and engage in risky behaviors.

Autism and ADHD highlight the same overarching theme of extremes: Interoceptive cues can be overly intense or too weak. Both hypersensitivity and hyposensitivity pose unique challenges, emphasizing the importance of finding a balanced level of interoceptive awareness across physical health, mental health, and behavior.

## When Physical Health Disrupts the Body's Signals

Health problems themselves interfere with communication between the brain and body. Since many bodily systems—cardiovascular, gastrointestinal, hormonal, and immune—produce interoceptive signals, it's not surprising that illness or imbalance in any of these systems can disrupt this communication. In this section, we'll look at key examples of how health issues influence our interoceptive experiences.

### *Complications from Illness*

Studies show that certain health conditions, such as diabetes, can interfere with how we perceive and respond to signals from our bodies. Austin Matus and colleagues found that people with type 1 diabetes who have difficulty paying attention to their bodily cues are more likely to miss the early warning signs of low blood sugar. In particular, those who worry less about their bodily sensations and struggle to attend to them are more prone to overlooking these early signs and may be slower to take steps to manage them.[7] By contrast, people who are better at recognizing and responding to bodily cues tend to follow treatment recommendations more consistently, leading to better health outcomes.

Millions have suffered from long COVID and its impact on interoceptive communication. They commonly experience heart palpitations, breathlessness, fainting, and extreme fatigue. Their bodily sensations suddenly feel "noisy" and overwhelming. Christopher Burton and his team of researchers suggest that this may stem from damage or inflammation in the vagus nerve and the insular cortex.[8] As we learned earlier, both are crucial in processing internal signals.

Inflammation more broadly complicates mind–body communication and appears in many conditions beyond long COVID, including autoimmune disorders (such as IBS and rheumatoid arthritis), cardiovascular disease, asthma, chronic obstructive pulmonary disease (COPD), and diabetes. It sensitizes the vagus nerve,[9] often leading to what researchers call "sickness behaviors": fatigue, low mood, anxiety, and increased pain sensitivity. These health issues reduce the clarity of bodily signals, making it harder for the brain to interpret them accurately.

### *Vagus Nerve Compression*

The vagus nerve is often called the "powerhouse nerve" because it carries interoceptive messages from the body to the brain and supports many aspects of physical and emotional health. Unlike the spinal cord, which is protected by the vertebrae, the vagus nerve is more exposed, making it vulnerable to injuries from whiplash, concussions, or surgery. Interestingly, even poor posture can strain this nerve, harming interoceptive function and overall health.

*Tech neck* is a growing problem in our device-heavy society. Tilting the head forward for long periods puts extra pressure on neck muscles and joints, compresses spinal discs, and can gradually change the natural curve of the upper spine. Doctors are seeing more cases of these postural issues, and the effects may go beyond stiffness or pain. Over time, the ligaments and tissues that help stabilize the neck can become strained or overstretched, weakening the neck's support structures. When this happens, nearby nerves and blood vessels may also be affected, influencing signals traveling between the brain and body. Research on cervical instability suggests this can contribute to a wide range of symptoms, including indigestion, heartburn, rapid heartbeat, shortness of breath, increased stress, poor sleep, mood changes, migraines, tinnitus, and vertigo.[10]

Many of these symptoms reflect changes in the body's internal signaling systems. Because interoception is the process through which the brain listens to signals from the body, disruptions along these pathways—including those involving nerves such as the vagus nerve—can influence how those signals are sensed and interpreted. While these symptoms can arise from many factors, research reminds us that even everyday habits like how we hold our heads while using our phones can shape how clearly the body receives its signals.

### *The Gut–Brain Connection*

The gut is a surprisingly complex part of our interoceptive system. It includes the entire digestive tract and the vast community of microorganisms living within it. The brain and gut communicate continuously through nerves like the vagus nerve, as well as through hormones and chemicals produced by gut bacteria. Emotions such as stress or anxiety can directly influence gut function—and even alter the balance of bacteria inside it. This ongoing exchange, known as the *gut–brain axis*, affects not only physical health but also emotional well-being and mental health. Research across gastroenterology, psychology, and neuroscience is demonstrating how central this connection is to interoception and emotional regulation.[11]

The idea of "gut feelings" isn't new. The ancient Greeks used the word *splanchna* to describe internal organs like the stomach and intestines, believing they were the source of deep emotions such as fear, love, and compassion. Modern science indicates they may have been onto something. Beyond digestion, the gut sends powerful interoceptive signals—hunger, fullness, nausea—that shape how we feel and think.

The gut also acts as a sensory organ, constantly communicating with the brain through neural and chemical pathways. It's where many important neurotransmitters and hormones are produced. More than 80 percent of the body's serotonin—a key chemical involved in mood, sleep, and digestion—is generated in the intestines, largely with the help of beneficial gut bacteria.[12]

Our gut is home to a large ecosystem of microbes, including bacteria, fungi, and even viruses. In the average person's gut alone, there are more than a thousand species of bacteria.[13] Microbial ecologist Jake Robinson refers to them as our "invisible friends" because of their vital role in our health.[14] These microbes do more than aid digestion; they support gut health, facilitate communication between the gut and brain, and play a key role in shaping interoception. Researchers Michael Ganci and colleagues add that gut microbes influence how we feel and regulate our internal states by producing neurotransmitters like serotonin.[15]

Unfortunately, the balance of gut microbes can be disrupted—a state known as *dysbiosis*. This occurs when microbial diversity decreases and beneficial bacteria decline. Diet plays a major role, especially diets high in refined sugar and ultra-processed foods. Alcohol and certain medications, including antibiotics, can also disrupt this balance. As Ganci and team note, the typical Western-style diet can weaken immune function and promote inflammation, which is closely linked to conditions such as anxiety and depression.[16]

Stress also has a powerful impact on the gut. Chronic stress, in particular, can damage the microbiome and cause it to shift in harmful ways. When gut microbes fall out of balance, the brain has a harder time accurately interpreting signals from the gut. Because these microbes help shape mood, perception, and internal awareness, disruptions in the microbiome can affect both physical and emotional health.

## Summing Up Bottom-Up Disruptions

It's essential to recognize the many factors that shape how we perceive our internal signals, because mind and body are deeply connected. What happens in the body doesn't stay in the body—it affects our entire system. Diabetes, for example, isn't just about blood sugar; it also raises the risk of anxiety and depression. The bacteria in our gut don't simply aid digestion; they also influence mood and sleep. Even poor posture isn't only about sore shoulders—it can affect both physical and mental health. Physical issues and mental health challenges are often intertwined.

One of the most important discoveries in this area is the role of interoceptive processes. At the core of the mind–body connection is interoception—the main way the body and brain communicate.

That's why a holistic approach to health matters. Rather than focusing on isolated symptoms, we need to consider the whole person. When we understand how the body and brain influence each other, we gain more tools to care for ourselves, manage stress, address mental health concerns, and support healing. In a world marked by rising stress, illness, and mental health challenges, we need every tool available. Strengthening the mind–body connection is essential to overall well-being. Simply put, when interoceptive communication works better, so do we.

# 6

# How Thoughts Shape Interoception

If you're not convinced that thoughts can influence the body, consider the many documented cases of psychogenic illness—once called "mass hysteria." One striking example occurred in the early 1960s at a textile factory in the United States and became known as the "June Bug" outbreak. Employees began reporting symptoms such as dizziness, nausea, and vomiting. Rumors quickly spread that a mysterious insect was biting workers on the factory floor, and as concern grew, more employees fell ill. Eventually, sixty-two workers reported symptoms. When the Centers for Disease Control investigated, they found no insects or environmental causes. The most likely explanation was not a hidden pest but the powerful interaction between belief and body—an example of psychogenic illness in which sickness arises from belief itself.[1]

Any discussion of interoceptive miscommunication must consider how thoughts influence bodily sensations. If you're familiar with cognitive behavioral therapy (CBT), you've likely heard of *cognitive distortions*, or thinking errors—habitual ways the mind can warp reality. Maybe you've assumed something is wrong when a text goes unanswered, or fixated on a single critical comment despite abundant positive feedback. Some people even blame themselves for events beyond their control. Irrational thinking involves holding beliefs that are not supported by evidence or logic. Just because we think something doesn't make it true—even when our bodies respond as if it is. CBT helps people identify and challenge these distortions, which are closely linked to mental health conditions such as depression and anxiety.

Recall that interoception is a two-way system. The body sends signals to the brain, and the brain responds by sending messages back to the body. Our thought patterns directly shape this communication. Mass hysteria illustrates this process on a large scale, but it plays out in everyday situations as well. What's important to note is that how we think can significantly influence what happens in our bodies.

Here are some examples that hit closer to home. Have you ever noticed your heart racing at the thought of a looming deadline? Does your stomach churn at the thought of giving a presentation at work? Just *thinking* about certain situations can trigger symptoms like a racing pulse, nausea, or insomnia. How often have you stayed awake worrying about not being able to fall asleep? In all these cases, thought patterns can hijack the body, sometimes with consequences for both physical and mental health.

Exaggerated or irrational ways of thinking don't just cloud judgment—they disrupt the mind–body connection. However, thought patterns are only part of the story. We also need to consider how thoughts affect bodily sensations and how those sensations, in turn, shape thought processes. As always, it's a two-way street.

In a nutshell, distorted thought patterns and interoceptive processes are deeply intertwined. The way we think significantly influences how we feel in our bodies, and the way we experience our bodies shapes how we think. This dynamic is key to understanding both mental and physical health challenges. As you'll see, cognitive distortions show up across several dimensions of interoceptive awareness measured by the MAIA questionnaire.

Let's take a closer look at a few common cognitive distortions through the lens of interoception. You'll begin to see how thoughts can affect the body—and how these effects vary from person to person. It's another reminder of the diversity of interoceptive experience.

## Misinterpretation of Bodily Sensations

How we interpret bodily sensations matters. When people tend to catastrophize, ordinary body signals can easily be misread as signs of danger.[2] Sometimes intestinal discomfort is just gas, not a warning sign. A twitching eyelid is usually just that—a twitch, not a sign of brain cancer. Often, people misread benign sensations as evidence of anxiety or danger. In these cases, harmless bodily signs become things to worry about unnecessarily.

Accurate interoception relies on noticing what's happening in the body and correctly identifying it. When sensations are misinterpreted, it becomes harder to regulate reactions and emotions effectively. Over time, repeated misreadings can erode trust in bodily signals—an essential component of interoceptive awareness measured by the MAIA. After all, trusting the body becomes difficult when its messages are regularly mislabeled.

*When Lauren is tired from being an overly involved caregiver, she tells herself that resting is selfish.*

*Catherine lives under the weight of many "shoulds." With her high expectations for herself, she (incorrectly) interprets fatigue and pain as personal weakness.*

*Nearly every sensation triggers concern for Hailey. She misinterprets, catastrophizes, and overgeneralizes many of her internal cues.*

*Ava worries about occasional bloating and water retention, viewing them as problems. So she pushes herself to exercise more and eat less.*

*Jason misreads sensations of hunger and irritation. When he gets hangry, he attributes his feelings to external causes—someone or something is making him feel upset—and uses that belief to justify his anger.*

*David views his bodily sensations through a self-critical, hopeless lens. This deepens his withdrawal and reinforces his belief that he is incapable of change.*

## Patterns of Exaggerating or Minimizing

Here's the Goldilocks principle again. Bodily sensations give us vital information, but they're only useful if we understand what they mean. Distorted thinking can lead people to exaggerate or minimize what they notice. Someone with disordered eating, for example, might ignore hunger cues and convince themselves they aren't hungry. On the other hand, a person with health anxiety may overreact to a harmless physical sensation, like an itch, which only heightens their discomfort.

The ability to recognize and correctly interpret bodily signals is central to the mind–body connection and to overall well-being. The brain does not simply read these signals—it predicts and interprets them. When those predictions are shaped by worry, catastrophic thinking, or past experiences, ordinary sensations can be misread. For example, everyday digestive discomfort may be mistaken for illness.[3]

*Roland downplays nearly all his bodily cues, whether they relate to emotions, physical needs, or health concerns.*

*Catherine also minimizes her need for rest and self-care, believing her needs are less important than those of others.*

*Lauren, by contrast, reads too much into her fatigue and bowel discomfort when she's emotionally overwhelmed, and this only increases her distress.*

*David's depression has narrowed his focus to a constant awareness of low energy. He feels so stuck that he can't even bring himself to make small changes that might help him feel better.*

Prediction errors are not the problem; they are opportunities for learning. Difficulties arise when the brain cannot, or does not, update its expectations in response to what the body is trying to communicate.

## Distortion of Emotional Experiences

Thought patterns also influence how emotions are experienced. The beliefs people hold about emotions—whether they are acceptable, controllable, or dangerous—can shape how those emotions are perceived and managed. Rigid or distorted thinking can alter emotional experience by influencing how feelings are interpreted. For example, black-and-white beliefs about emotions like anger or sadness may lead someone to see them as entirely good or entirely bad. Beliefs such as *Men don't cry* or *Anger is always unhealthy* can prevent people from acknowledging what they feel.

When someone believes it's wrong to feel a certain way, they may suppress or dismiss the emotion. But emotions are also experienced through physical changes in the body. When people push emotions away, they may also ignore the bodily signals that accompany them, weakening emotional awareness and making regulation harder. After all, we cannot manage an emotion we've convinced ourselves we aren't feeling—or one we assume is completely justified regardless of the situation.

*Roland dismisses the validity of emotions altogether. He strongly favors what he considers "rational thinking." He believes emotions are for the weak and the unintelligent.*

*Jason believes that, as a man, anger is the only acceptable emotion. He externalizes blame for his anger and never takes responsibility for it.*

*Hailey assumes that because she feels anxious, something must be wrong. She also interprets emotional sensations as signs of illness.*

*David's catastrophic thinking deepens his hopelessness and despair. He believes nothing will ever improve for him or his family—a thought pattern that fuels his worry.*

## Discounting the Positive and Focusing on the Negative

We all know someone who seems to put a negative spin on everything. Applied to interoception, this pattern shows up as a tendency to focus excessively on what feels uncomfortable, painful, or anxiety-provoking in the body. This fixed attention on the negative makes it easy to overlook pleasant sensations like comfort, relaxation, or enjoyment. In time, awareness increasingly locks onto bodily discomfort until that's primarily what a person notices.

This negative filter is especially common among people living with chronic pain or panic disorder.[4] Shifting attention away from discomfort isn't easy, but it's essential for well-being. Focusing persistently on pain or tension not only crowds out signals of ease but also makes it harder to develop a healthy connection with the body. Eventually, this pattern contributes to the distressing symptoms in many of the conditions explored in Part 3 of this book.

*Catherine strongly feels she hasn't done enough or worked hard enough, and she constantly searches for ways to push herself.*

*Lauren tends to expect the worst from her decisions, which fuels her anxiety and leads to analysis paralysis.*

*David's catastrophizing and rumination deepen his emotional distress. All-or-nothing thinking contributes to his belief that he's a failure, preventing him from enjoying time with his family or engaging in hobbies he once found meaningful.*

## Excessive Worry About Sensation

Some people become overly anxious when they experience physical discomfort, such as indigestion or muscle tension. Rather than staying calm, they ruminate on these sensations—a pattern research shows can intensify the perception of symptoms and worsen discomfort.[5]

We know that interoception is a two-way system: The body sends signals to the brain, and the brain responds in turn. When distorted thoughts feed into this loop, they amplify the very sensations that sparked the worry. For example, someone with social anxiety may fear that others will notice their sweating or trembling at a party. The thought *Everyone is staring at me* heightens their anxiety, which increases the symptoms. Those stronger sensations then feel like confirmation of the fear, reinforcing avoidance of social situations.

*Ava is acutely sensitive to sensations she associates with physical attractiveness. Her fear of gaining weight drives her to overexercise and severely restrict her food intake. Unfortunately, the physical stress this creates increases her emotional distress, which exacerbates her anxiety about her appearance.*

*Hailey's intense awareness of bodily sensations, combined with her tendency to imagine the worst, turns small, harmless signals into perceived threats. This fuels a cycle of health anxiety, leading her to constantly monitor her body, feel panicked, and seek reassurance.*

*David tends to interpret sensations as signs of personal failure; even minor discomfort can feel overwhelming. His catastrophizing exaggerates these sensations, turning normal bodily cues into sources of distress. Over time, this cycle deepens his feelings of inadequacy, leaving him more depressed and withdrawn.*

## Prediction Errors Revisited

Now that we've looked at how cognitive distortions influence interoception, let's return to the concept of predictive processing introduced in Chapter 2. Researchers such as Lisa Feldman Barrett and Karen Quigley have highlighted the role of predictive processing in interoceptive experience and the brain's interpretation of bodily signals.[6] The brain doesn't merely respond to signals from the body; it actively predicts what the body should be feeling. This means our internal experiences are shaped by what our brain expects to feel. Pause for a moment and let that sink in: What we feel internally is strongly influenced by what the brain believes *should* be happening.

The earlier example of drinking water when thirsty illustrates this process. Long before water has actually hydrated the body, thirst is often relieved. That's predictive processing at work: The brain anticipates that the water will meet the body's hydration needs, so it reduces the thirst sensation before hydration levels have actually changed. Sometimes, however, the brain's expectation doesn't align with reality, and we encounter a *prediction error*. Ideally, the brain updates its prediction in response to this mismatch. But this type of learning becomes harder when cognitive distortions are widespread. Instead of correcting the error, distorted thinking tends to reinforce it.

A healthy interoceptive process depends on updating predictions when they are wrong. Here are some examples of what this looks like:

PAIN PERCEPTION

**Prediction:** My knee will be fine if I go for a run.

**Actual Signal:** Sharp pain when moving the knee after an injury.

**Updated Prediction:** I should stop running. My knee probably isn't healed yet.

**Prediction Error:** Oh, it's nothing. I'll be fine, leading to continued running and a worsened injury.

EMOTIONAL CUES

**Prediction:** This will be easy. I won't get frustrated putting this shelf together.

**Actual Signals:** Racing heart, sweating, growing irritation.

**Updated Prediction:** This is harder than I expected. I should take a break.

**Prediction Error:** I'm not annoyed. I'm fine, which clearly isn't true, given the signs of frustration—swearing and throwing tools included.

ANXIETY RESPONSE

**Prediction:** Talking to this person will be terrifying. My anxiety will be really high.

**Actual Signals:** Staying relatively calm; the interaction feels smooth.

**Updated Prediction:** It wasn't that bad. I don't need to be so afraid.

**Prediction Error:** I got lucky this time. Next time my anxiety will be worse—a belief that keeps anxiety elevated in future interactions.

As seen in many interoception-related processes, predictions can follow an over- or underestimation pattern. In the prior examples, task-related pain and emotional challenges were underestimated, while the anticipated anxiety of a social interaction was overestimated.

Many mental health challenges—anxiety in particular—involve predictions that overestimate negative outcomes. People tend to perceive danger where there is none. For instance, someone with anxiety or panic disorder might interpret their symptoms and sensations as far more serious than they are. A similar pattern can occur in some pain conditions, where sensations become amplified because the individual overestimates how intense the pain is. These patterns often lead to hypervigilance and catastrophizing bodily signals, which can increase emotional instability, fear, and distress.

Conversely, some people tend to underestimate their internal cues. This is common in depression and certain eating disorders, where awareness of bodily sensations—such as emotions or hunger—is diminished. These individuals' responses often involve numbing or ignoring bodily cues altogether.

When prediction errors aren't updated, the brain continues to trust its original prediction. Let's look at how some of the people we've been following experience prediction errors that follow over- or underestimation patterns.

*Roland consistently underestimates his body's signals, insisting he's "fine" despite clear signs to the contrary, including acid reflux, emotional disconnection, and a strained marriage. He overlooks early health warnings and remains emotionally numb to his wife's concerns, convinced that everything is under control—even when it isn't.*

*Catherine believes she should have the energy to do everything. She ignores hunger, fatigue, and stress, pushing herself to meet every expectation. Rather than adjusting her beliefs to include rest and nourishment, she dismisses these bodily cues as weakness.*

*For Jason, prediction errors fuel anger, impulsivity, and drinking alcohol. Since he views any emotion other than anger as weakness, he dismisses them or reinterprets them as anger. He automatically assumes he's being disrespected or threatened whenever his bodily sensations increase, making him quick to explode and act impulsively.*

*Hailey overestimates the threat associated with bodily sensations. Even harmless cues are interpreted as signs of imminent danger—her brain insists that a racing heart means she's about to faint. Reassurance from doctors or family doesn't change these beliefs, leaving her caught in a cycle of anxiety driven by persistent prediction errors and heightened fear.*

## Comparing Cognitive Distortions and Predictive Processing

At first glance, cognitive distortions and predictive processing may seem quite similar. Both involve errors in perception or interpretation. Both can generate self-reinforcing loops, just in different ways. And both can increase anxiety and distress.

Despite these surface similarities, the differences between the two are far more significant. Cognitive distortions involve the content of our thoughts. They are habitual patterns of thinking that misinterpret reality from a mental perspective. While this chapter primarily focuses on cognitive distortions that influence how we perceive bodily cues, irrational thought patterns can also show up in personal areas, such as relationships or job performance. These patterns are not limited to bodily processes.

By contrast, predictive processing is a theory about how the brain works. Remember, the brain makes predictions about all incoming sensory information to improve efficiency. This process is fundamental to how humans operate and usually happens unconsciously. Prediction errors occur when there's a mismatch between what the brain expects and what actually happens. Problems arise when those errors aren't updated and corrected.

At the same time, cognitive distortions and predictive processing can feed into each other in ways that amplify emotional distress and mental health challenges. Predictive processing explains how the brain manages mismatches between expectation and reality; cognitive distortions are the stories we tell ourselves about those mismatches. When distorted thought patterns take hold, they prevent the brain from revising its predictions in light of new information. For example, when Catherine interprets fatigue as weakness, her cognitive distortions keep her brain from recognizing that her bodily needs matter. This kind of thinking locks the error in place instead of allowing the brain to correct it. When both processes are active, they reinforce each other, perpetuating a negative cycle.

# 7

# The Influence of Early Attachments

You may recall stories about young animals forming strong bonds, or imprinting, on humans or even other species. Imprinting is the powerful social bond a young animal forms, most often with its parent. Occasionally, however, this process is disrupted, causing the animal to bond with something else instead. It's not uncommon to hear of birds such as ducks or geese imprinting on humans and following them around. There are also striking examples of cross-species imprinting, including baby antelopes cuddling with a lioness in Kenya and a marmoset in Brazil clinging to a capuchin monkey.[1]

Imprinting is an instinctive process that helps animals survive. It enables young animals to identify members of their species and learn essential survival skills. Human infants undergo a similar—though far more complex—social bonding process known as *attachment*. While imprinting happens quickly and instinctually, attachment develops gradually as babies form expectations about safety, care, and connection. Importantly, attachment isn't just emotional—it is a biological necessity.

Just as imprinting helps young animals connect with what keeps them alive, human infants rely on a neurobiological system designed to seek safety through connection. Babies depend on caregivers not only for food and protection but also for *co-regulation*—attuned interactions that help regulate and stabilize an infant's physical and emotional states.

## Co-Regulation: The Biological Foundation of Attachment

Drawing on the work of clinician and neuroscientist Allan Schore, early attachment is primarily a process of learning how to regulate emotions within relationships. An infant's nervous system is not yet developed enough to handle stress on its own. From the very beginning of life, babies depend on caregivers to help organize their internal states.[2]

Long before language develops, infants respond to tone of voice, facial expressions, eye contact, rhythm, and touch. These cues communicate safety and help settle the body. When caregivers are warm, responsive, and soothing, they reduce distress and support recovery from stress. Over time, through thousands of small interactions, the child's ability to regulate emotions begins to take shape.

Babies cannot soothe themselves at first. They learn to settle by repeatedly experiencing comfort. When an infant is rocked, spoken to softly, and held warmly, the caregiver is doing more than offering comfort; they are helping the child's body learn what calmness feels like. With consistency, these comforting moments gradually shape how the child manages intense emotions, recovers from stress, and understands what is happening inside their body.

When caregiving is inconsistent, frightening, or emotionally distant, calming down becomes harder. Without steady support, a child might become easily overwhelmed or turn inward and shut down. These early patterns can influence how safe the world feels, what the child expects from others, and how they perceive themselves.

Simply put, attachment begins with biology. Experiences of co-regulation form the basis for emotional resilience, social trust, and interoceptive awareness—the capacity to sense and understand what is happening inside the body. These early regulatory patterns later underpin what attachment theory describes as *attachment styles*.

## Attachment Theory

Attachment theory, first developed by John Bowlby in the mid-1900s, explains how early bonds with caregivers shape emotional and social development across the lifespan. Bowlby proposed that infants are biologically wired to seek closeness to caregivers—especially in times of stress—not just for physical survival but also for emotional security.[3] These early experiences lay the groundwork for how we learn to trust, connect with others, and regulate our emotions.[4]

Mary Ainsworth later expanded on Bowlby's work by identifying core attachment styles: secure, insecure-ambivalent, and insecure-avoidant.[5] In discussions of adult attachment, the term *anxious* is typically used in place of *ambivalent*, reflecting a persistent worry about relationships.

*Secure attachment* forms when infants receive consistent, responsive care. In the long term, they come to feel safe and protected, trusting that their needs will be met with kindness. Their bodies also learn a crucial skill: how to move from states of activation or distress back into calm. In contrast, insecure attachment occurs when caregivers are emotionally unavailable, inconsistent, or overly intrusive. In many cases, caregivers face challenges that hinder their ability to provide a secure base, including stress, trauma, mental health concerns, or their own attachment histories.

Social inequity creates additional barriers to attachment and co-regulation. When caregivers live with poverty, racism, unsafe neighborhoods, or chronic time scarcity, their capacity to provide consistent care is often limited—not because of a lack of care or good intentions but due to ongoing stress from systemic pressures. Housing instability, food insecurity, unpredictable work schedules, and discrimination all make emotional availability harder to sustain. In these situations, infants may receive care that is loving but inconsistent, attentive yet intermittently unavailable, as caregivers manage exhaustion and persistent stressors.

*Insecure attachment* typically presents in two primary ways: People with an *anxious attachment* style often worry about rejection or abandonment. They may dislike being alone, seek frequent reassurance, and struggle with feelings of unworthiness. On the other hand, those with *avoidant attachment* tend to find closeness uncomfortable, place a high value on independence, and downplay emotional needs. Both attachment styles reflect how early experiences of regulation organize expectations about safety, connection, and distress. Early relationships shape our attachment patterns, whether secure, anxious, or avoidant. These patterns, in turn, shape how we manage emotions, cope with stress, build relationships, and see ourselves in the world.

## The Attachment–Interoception Connection

From birth onward, infants rely entirely on their caregivers—not just for food and safety, but also for comfort, regulation, and help making sense of their internal world. Babies don't come into the world knowing whether they're hungry, tired, or scared. When these sensations arise, all they register is that something feels wrong. Through a caregiver's response—feeding them when they're hungry, soothing them when they're upset, and putting words to their experiences—babies start to link body sensations with meaning. Caregivers translate internal states into language: "You're hungry," "That scared you," or "Ouch, that must have hurt." In time, these interactions help infants begin to understand their inner world.

Interoception does not develop in isolation. Psychologist Kristina Oldroyd and her colleagues emphasize that for children to truly understand their bodies, caregivers must acknowledge their experiences and reflect them back. Oldroyd offers the example of a toddler who falls while learning to walk. A caregiver saying, "Ouch! That must have hurt," supports the child's developing interoceptive awareness. In contrast, a response like "You're fine! That didn't hurt. Get back up!" invalidates the child's internal cues and interferes with the learning process.[6]

When caregivers name sensations, soothe distress, and remain emotionally present, the child's nervous system learns that their inner experience matters and that their feelings can be trusted. But when caregivers minimize, dismiss, or ignore bodily cues, children learn the opposite: that their sensations are confusing, unreliable, and unimportant. In time, this can disrupt interoceptive awareness and contribute to emotional and relational difficulties later in life. The key point is that attachment provides the relational pathway through which interoceptive awareness develops.

## How Attachment Styles Shape Interoception

Secure attachment helps build a flexible, trusting relationship with bodily cues. When caregivers consistently provide warm, responsive care, children learn to recognize and trust their internal signals. In everyday moments—feeding a fussy baby, comforting them to sleep—caregivers help children connect their body sensations with meaning. These interactions also help build emotional regulation. Babies aren't born knowing how to manage strong feelings—any toddler's meltdown makes that clear. But attentive, sensitive caregivers act as external regulators, helping children navigate overwhelming emotions. Supportive parenting equips them with tools for managing stress and feelings as they grow.[7] Securely attached children also develop flexible nervous systems capable of shifting between states of activation and calm, and they become increasingly skilled at making sense of their internal experiences.

Insecure attachment disrupts this process. When physical or emotional needs are not consistently met, children may learn that their internal signals do not matter. If a child is not fed when hungry or is told "nothing's wrong" when clearly upset, they may begin to doubt or ignore bodily sensations, leading to confusion about needs, emotions, and bodily awareness.

Oldroyd and colleagues found that anxiously attached individuals report noticing more bodily sensations, having greater emotional awareness, and—most notably—worrying significantly more about what those sensations imply.[8] This pattern reflects a state of chronic sympathetic activation or mobilization, in which the nervous system remains on high alert, constantly scanning for potential threats.

Avoidant attachment involves distancing oneself from bodily cues. Oldroyd and colleagues found that individuals with this pattern tend to pay less attention to bodily sensations and trust them less, often suppressing negative feelings before they fully register.[9]

In both cases, children adapt to the caregiving they receive, but these adaptations can cause lasting difficulties with body awareness and emotional processing. As authors Daniel Siegel and Mary Hartzell point out, it's especially confusing when a child's reality is denied by the very people they depend on most.[10] What begins as a survival strategy in childhood can continue to shape how the body and brain communicate for years to come.

## How Attachment Impacts the Developing Brain

An infant's brain is still developing, and the early years are especially crucial for establishing the foundations of healthy brain function. The bond between a child and their caregiver influences not only emotional development but also the brain circuits involved in interoception—particularly the insular cortex, the hub for processing internal signals.[11] Studies show that babies begin to show awareness of bodily sensations as early as five months,[12] highlighting how quickly these systems develop and how strongly they rely on caregiving relationships. When caregivers are warm, consistent, and attentive, they create a sense of safety that fosters secure attachment, healthy brain development, and effective interoceptive awareness.

In contrast, insecure attachment can interfere with the maturation of brain structures that help children interpret bodily cues and regulate emotions. Researchers increasingly describe emotionally or physically unresponsive caregiving as a form of early relational trauma.[13] A review of studies on attachment, eating disorders, and self-harm found that individuals with eating disorders often show changes in the insula and other interoceptive brain regions—areas strongly shaped by early caregiving.[14] When caregivers fail to provide reliable food or comfort, the brain may learn to interpret bodily signals inconsistently, weakening the link between sensation and emotion.

## How Insecure Attachment Shows Up in Adulthood

Our earliest relationships inform how we perceive our emotions, connect with others, and listen to our bodies. Adults who received consistent, responsive caregiving often develop a stable internal blueprint: They can trust others, interpret bodily cues accurately, and use interoceptive signals to manage both their bodily functions and emotions. As children, their nervous system learned that distress could be soothed and that connection was generally safe. For adults with insecure attachment, these processes are often more difficult. Defensive nervous system states learned in childhood—highly activated or shutdown—do not disappear. They continue to shape how individuals sense their bodies, regulate emotions, and relate to others.

### *Anxious Attachment*

Adults with anxious attachment often experience heightened awareness and sensitivity to bodily sensations.[15] Because comfort and attunement were inconsistent in childhood, their nervous system learned to stay on alert, constantly scanning for signs of relational or bodily danger. Research by Oldroyd and colleagues shows that anxiously attached individuals tend to notice bodily sensations more intensely (hyperawareness), react more strongly to them, worry about what they might mean, and struggle to use bodily cues to guide effective emotion regulation.[16] In other words, their bodies behave just as their attachment system does: vigilant, activated, and anxious.

Since anxious attachment increases the misinterpretation of bodily signals, it can lead to anxiety and rumination, which further contribute to emotional instability. People with this pattern often seek reassurance from others because they lack trust in their ability to interpret their body's messages. In short, someone with anxious attachment tends to overfocus on internal signals, worry excessively about them, struggle to use bodily cues for insight, and have reduced trust in their bodily sensations—several of the MAIA dimensions affected by anxious attachment. You will see why these patterns developed for Lauren and Hailey.

*Lauren grew up with a mom who had Multiple Sclerosis (MS), so she took on a caregiving role as a teenager. She learned to set her own needs aside to avoid adding stress to the family, forming the belief that her worth depended on caring for others. As an adult, she continues to put others first at the cost of her own health and energy. While she is very sensitive to those around her, this pattern leaves her anxious, exhausted, and hesitant to seek support for fear of being a burden.*

***Hailey's anxious attachment style was shaped by early food intolerances and her mother's close monitoring of her symptoms and diet. Although her mother's care was well-intentioned, it reinforced the belief that Hailey's body was fragile and needed constant attention. Hailey learned to pay very close attention to her sensations and to seek reassurance from others to feel safe. Even though her intolerances are now well managed, this pattern persists into adulthood, showing up as health anxiety, overanalyzing symptoms, and frequent reassurance-seeking.***

## *Avoidant Attachment*

Research suggests that attachment patterns influence how people relate to their internal bodily signals. Individuals with anxious attachment often become highly attuned to physical cues linked to distress, while those with avoidant attachment tend to move in the opposite direction. Rather than leaning into their internal experiences, avoidantly attached individuals are more likely to minimize or suppress bodily signals.[17] By pushing these cues out of awareness, they avoid sensations that might feel overwhelming or emotionally vulnerable. In this way, their attachment style shows up in the body as a defensive shutdown—an attempt to stay safe by not feeling too much.

Over time, this coping style can shape how much attention people give to their internal cues. Studies show that the more avoidant a person's attachment style, the less attention they pay to their bodily sensations and the less they tend to trust those signals. As a result, there can be a disconnect between what someone says they feel and what their body is actually experiencing.[18] A person may insist they are not angry or stressed even when their heart rate, muscle tension, or other physiological markers suggest otherwise. Avoidantly attached individuals may even appear calm during stressful situations while their physiological stress responses remain elevated.[19]

When people habitually minimize or suppress their body's signals, important information about their internal state can be missed. They may overlook early signs of stress, fatigue, or emotional strain, making it harder to recognize when they need rest, support, or a change in direction. Eventually, this reduced awareness can contribute to difficulties with emotional regulation, delayed responses to stress or illness, and a growing sense of disconnection from their own internal experience.

MAIA scores for avoidantly attached individuals show reduced interoceptive awareness across multiple dimensions, including their ability to notice internal sensations, connect bodily cues to emotions, regulate emotional and behavioral responses, and trust bodily signals. Roland and Ava's childhood experiences illustrate why these patterns develop.

*Roland grew up with parents who survived World War II in Europe before relocating to the United States. They worked hard to create a stable life but rarely showed emotion or affection. Without the warmth he needed, Roland learned it was safer to rely on himself, stay busy, and avoid depending on others. As an adult, he keeps people at arm's length, focusing on work and routines instead of feelings. He struggles to recognize or express emotions, leaving him distant from his family and disconnected from both his inner world and his body's signals.*

*Ava was raised in a wealthy household with busy executive parents, so much of her care came from nannies. Although her material needs were met, she lacked consistent emotional support. She learned to seek comfort and identity through her appearance and external approval. As a young adult, she maintains shallow or transactional relationships, struggles to trust others, and is highly reactive to criticism or perceived neglect.*

## It's Never Too Late to Learn

When exploring the challenges someone faced as a child, it helps to remember that the goal is to understand what shaped their interoceptive awareness, not to assign blame. It's about identifying the impact of our early experiences so that healing pathways can emerge. Seeing how closely attachment and interoception are linked makes it clear why early experiences matter so much. For some, this can be a painful realization; many caregivers simply lacked the resources or awareness to offer consistent connection and support.

But there is hope. Interoceptive awareness isn't fixed. Our ability for safe, connected relationships can develop throughout life. Relational skills can be strengthened, interoception can become clearer, and emotional flexibility can be restored. These abilities can be improved at any age, leading to resilience and greater well-being.

# 8

# Understanding the Stress Response

In the opening chapter of *Why Zebras Don't Get Ulcers*, a fascinating book on neuroscience by Dr. Robert Sapolsky, the author highlights a striking point: "Our current patterns of disease would be unrecognizable to our great-grandparents or, for that matter, to most mammals."[1] In the late 1800s, the leading causes of premature death were infectious diseases like influenza and tuberculosis, complications of childbirth, and accidents.

Today, that list looks very different. Thanks to vaccinations and modern medicine, the risks associated with infectious disease and childbirth have dramatically decreased. Instead, the most common causes of death now include heart disease, cancer, stroke, chronic respiratory diseases like COPD, and diabetes. Sapolsky links many of these modern conditions to a subtle but persistent factor: chronic stress.

Sapolsky also notes that zebras (and other wild animals) face acute stressors—escaping a predator, competing for resources, and surviving in the wild. Their stress response is intense but short-lived. Once the threat passes, their bodies return to baseline. The stress response does what it was designed to do: mobilize energy for survival and then shut off.[2]

Humans, however, can activate these same biological stress responses not because of immediate physical danger but because of ongoing pressures—work demands, finances, relationships, uncertainty, or worries about the future. Unlike the short bursts of stress animals experience, these pressures can keep the body's stress systems partially active for extended periods. Over time, this prolonged activation strains multiple body systems and contributes to many of the health problems we see today.

At the center of this process is the autonomic nervous system (ANS)—the network that regulates heart rate, breathing, digestion, blood pressure, and many other automatic functions that quietly keep us alive. The ANS is not simply reacting to physical threats; it is constantly adjusting the body in response to how the brain interprets what is happening around us and within us.

Stress is more than just a thought. It is also a bodily experience, involving interoceptive processes such as shifts in heart rhythm, muscle tension, breathing, hormone release, and inflammation. Understanding these bodily reactions is essential for distinguishing between acute and chronic stress, and for recognizing the long-term effects of chronic stress on our health and well-being.

## What Is the Stress Response?

Our stress response begins the moment the brain detects a threat or stressor. That threat can be real—like an approaching deadline—or imagined, such as worrying about being fired without cause. It may be significant, for instance a car accident, or minor, such as hearing a sudden loud noise. The amygdala helps identify potential threats and activates the stress response; it functions much like a smoke alarm.

The stress response triggered by the amygdala is often called the *fight-or-flight response*. When a threat is perceived, the amygdala initiates a series of reactions involving multiple systems in the body. In general, the stress response unfolds in the following sequence:

1. **Threat detection:** The amygdala senses danger and signals the hypothalamus to activate the stress response.
2. **System activation:** The hypothalamus alerts two systems—the sympathetic-adrenal-medullary (SAM) system and the hypothalamic-pituitary-adrenal (HPA) axis.
3. **Immediate response:** The SAM system kicks in first, triggering the classic "fight or flight" response. Adrenaline is released within seconds, speeding up heart rate and breathing while redirecting blood flow from digestion to the muscles. This gives the body a quick burst of energy to face the threat.
4. **Sustained response:** The HPA axis activates alongside the SAM system but with a slower, longer-lasting response. It releases cortisol, which keeps the stress response going when the initial energy boost isn't enough. Cortisol raises blood sugar for sustained energy but suppresses functions like immunity, digestion, and reproduction

to conserve resources. In essence, the body says: *Survive now; handle everything else later.*

5. **Recovery:** Once the threat has passed, the parasympathetic nervous system (PNS) activates the "rest and digest" response. Heart rate and breathing slow, muscles relax, and systems like digestion and immunity resume normal functioning as the body returns to baseline.

When this recovery phase doesn't occur, the stress response lingers and can shift into chronic stress. And as we'll see, certain situations can delay recovery. Zebras don't get ulcers because once the chase ends, their bodies return to normal quickly. Humans, however, can remain stuck in a heightened stress response with high cortisol levels for extended periods. That's where the real damage begins.

Before going further, it helps to define what a *stressor* is. In simple terms, it's anything that adds pressure to our system. It doesn't matter whether this trigger is physical, emotional, or psychological; the body's stress response is remarkably similar. Almost getting in a car accident, a tough exam, or even anticipating a big presentation can activate it. That's the human twist: Unlike zebras, we don't need a predator chasing us to feel stressed. Just thinking about money issues, relationship conflicts, or "what if" scenarios about the future can activate the same physiological response.

The real challenge is chronic stress—the kind that lingers. Financial strain, toxic workplaces, painful relationships, long-term insomnia, or lack of social support can keep the stress response turned on for weeks, months, or even years. Our bodies aren't designed for such prolonged activation. Add modern lifestyle factors, such as poor diet, sleep deprivation, alcohol or drug use, and habits like doom-scrolling, and the strain intensifies.

Animals don't face these problems. They don't worry about tomorrow's food supply, eat processed snacks, or lie awake scrolling on their phones. Nor do they contend with mortgages or navigate the stress of keeping up with modern technology. They experience stress in the moment and then recover. That's why, as Sapolsky notes, zebras don't get ulcers—but we do.

## Our Body Under Pressure

Turning on our stress response isn't all bad. In fact, it is essential for survival because it helps us respond to threats and dangerous situations. It can even boost motivation and enhance performance when stress is short-term and manageable. The problem arises when stress becomes chronic, driven by anticipatory fears, psychological stressors, lifestyle choices, and other factors. When we're under long-term stress, our health and mental well-being take a serious hit. Here are some ways chronic stress and excess cortisol negatively impact key bodily functions.

**Cardiovascular and respiratory systems.** During stress, breathing and blood pressure rise to quickly deliver oxygen and energy to the muscles for fight or flight. But when blood pressure stays elevated for too long, it strains the heart and blood vessels, increasing the risk of heart disease, heart attack, and stroke. Common symptoms include a rapid heartbeat, palpitations, shortness of breath, dizziness, and high blood pressure.

**Gastrointestinal system.** Stress disrupts digestion by diverting blood away from the gut and slowing its normal processes. This can reduce digestive secretions, change how food moves through the intestines, and disturb gut bacteria. The results often include nausea, heartburn, bloating, constipation, or diarrhea.

**Muscular system.** Stress causes muscles to tense as part of the fight-or-flight response. When stress persists, that tension lingers and leads to soreness and pain, especially in the neck, jaw, and lower back. It's also a common trigger for stress-related headaches.

**Endocrine (hormonal) systems.** Chronic stress and high cortisol disrupt hormonal balance. Cortisol raises blood sugar and can lead to weight gain, particularly around the abdomen, which increases the risk of type 2 diabetes. It also interferes with reproductive hormones, causing cycle changes, fertility issues, or premenstrual syndrome (PMS) in women and lowering testosterone and sperm count in men.

**Immune system.** Long-term stress weakens immunity, leaving us more vulnerable to infections such as colds and cold sores. It also increases inflammation throughout the body and contributes to autoimmune disorders such as lupus, chronic fatigue syndrome, arthritis, and fibromyalgia.

**Sleep patterns.** Stress and sleep are uneasy partners. Racing thoughts and a wired-up nervous system make it harder to fall asleep, while stress dreams or 3 a.m. wakeups keep us from staying asleep. The less rest we get, the more stressed we feel, creating a vicious cycle.

Did you notice that many of the systems affected by stress are the same ones that generate interoceptive sensations? In other words, stress hijacks the very signals we depend on for our well-being. And often, we don't even realize it's happening. When you compare the systems impacted by stress with those that produce interoceptive cues, the overlap is striking. It's a powerful reminder that stress engages many of our major bodily systems. Even when stress is emotional or psychological, it still affects the entire body.

And it's important to remember that interoceptive signals reflect the constant activity happening inside us. They are responsible for many functions, including regulating bodily processes, shaping our emotions, and strengthening our social connections. But when chronic stress keeps "jacking up" these systems, each of those areas suffers. That's why managing stress isn't just about feeling calmer—it's about protecting the very processes that keep us connected to ourselves and to others.

## Chronic Stress and Interoceptive Disturbances

Ever notice how some people snap more easily when they're stressed? We've all seen someone overreact to something small, like being cut off in traffic or a barista getting their order wrong. Chances are, it's not really about the latte. What's more likely is that their body is stuck in fight-or-flight mode. Chronic stress keeps the system *on*, which messes with how a person experiences and interprets their internal signals.

During stress, a feedback loop can kick in: Sensations like a racing heart or shortness of breath can feel more intense. When those sensations cause distress, they raise stress levels even further and keep the stress response going.[3] We're also more likely to misinterpret what we feel, which creates even more stress. Over time, this blurs our ability to read our bodies accurately. It also makes it harder to read situations, increasing the likelihood of overreacting to a perceived threat. When someone is stuck in a chronic fight-or-flight state, they are more likely to sense harm or danger where none exists.

Research shows that interoceptive awareness can make a big difference here. Roberta Allegretta and colleagues found that people who are better at noticing and managing their internal signals handle stress with more clarity and emotional balance.[4] Being able to recognize when we're having a stress-induced emotional response is helpful; being able to practice healthy coping strategies in those moments is even better.

But the flip side is also true. When our interoceptive awareness is low, we're not tuned in, and we may not even realize we're in a stress response. Instead, we assume the problem is "out there"—the barista, the traffic, the email from a colleague. Add in our culture of distraction—scrolling, drinking, anything to avoid feeling discomfort—and stress festers. The less we notice it, the worse our regulation gets, and the more likely we are to explode over small things.

That's why interoceptive skills matter so much. Learning to notice stress cues and use them to calm ourselves can interrupt the cycle of chronic stress. Imagine if more of us could do this—spotting the signs early, responding with steadiness, and stopping stress from spilling onto others. It would make the world a kinder place, simply by paying closer attention to our bodily cues. Improving interoceptive awareness not only benefits our health but also strengthens our connections with those around us. And honestly, the world could use more of that right now.

## All the Stresses—What's the Difference?

We use the word *stress* a lot, but it carries different nuances depending on the situation. We've already explored what stress is and how chronic stress affects the body. But what about traumatic stress and post-traumatic stress disorder (PTSD)? These terms can be confusing, so it helps to break them down. All types of stress trigger the same physiological systems and responses we've already covered, but they differ in intensity, impact, and duration.

**Stress.** Stress is the body's normal response to everyday challenges. It can be physical, emotional, or psychological. Sometimes, it's even positive, like feeling excited before a big presentation or a new adventure. Other times it's negative, such as arguing with a coworker or getting stuck in traffic. Stress responses are usually short-term: They activate when the stressor appears and subside once it's gone. Not all stress is harmful; in fact, it can sometimes help us perform better in challenging situations.

**Chronic stress.** Problems arise when stress becomes persistent. Ongoing, long-term challenges—financial struggles, social inequities, discrimination, single parenting, caring for a sick loved one, or being in an unhealthy relationship—keep stress hormones elevated. Unlike wild animals that return to a nonstressed state after escaping a predator, humans often stay "switched on" in a chronic stress state. Eventually, this constant surge of cortisol takes a toll on both mind and body, raising the risk of physical illness and mental health difficulties.

**Traumatic stress.** Traumatic stress is different in both intensity and impact. Trauma refers to events involving actual or perceived danger that is significantly more severe or life-threatening than everyday stressors, such as natural disasters, accidents, abuse, or assaults. These experiences activate the same stress response as everyday stress but at a much higher level. The feelings of fear, horror, or helplessness that come from trauma make its effects far more profound.

Recovery from traumatic stress takes longer than recovery from everyday stress. It takes time and support for the nervous system to settle following a traumatic event. It's normal to have nightmares, flashbacks, and overwhelming emotions in the days or weeks that follow. The good news is that healing is possible, and many people do recover with time and care.

**Post-traumatic stress disorder (PTSD).** PTSD is a mental health condition that can develop after a traumatic event. The key difference is duration and impact: Unlike typical stress reactions, PTSD symptoms don't fade within a few weeks. If they last more than a month and disrupt daily life, it may be PTSD. In simple terms, the body and brain remain stuck in fight-or-flight mode long after the danger is gone. People with PTSD often feel as if their stress response never turns off. They may live with a rapid heartbeat, shortness of breath, high blood pressure, muscle tension, stomach problems, poor sleep, and a constant sense of being on guard. Many also relive the trauma through nightmares or flashbacks. These symptoms can last for months or even years if left untreated.

We'll explore trauma and PTSD in much more depth in an upcoming chapter, as understanding their effects on interoceptive awareness warrants a fuller, dedicated discussion.

## How Chronic Stress Shows Up

To understand how chronic stress affects interoceptive awareness, coping mechanisms, and daily functioning, let's look at the individuals we've been following and how a constantly engaged fight-or-flight response shows up in their lives.

*Roland lives with chronic stress but insists he feels fine. He ignored his acid reflux until it caused damage and dismissed his wife's concerns about his blood pressure. Predictability and logic are his main coping tools—he keeps strict routines, overworks, and relies on problem-solving instead of emotional awareness. These strategies give him a sense of control but keep his stress response activated, reducing enjoyment and spontaneity and leaving him emotionally distant and disconnected from his body's signals.*

*Catherine is always busy. Even when her body needs rest, she pushes through, driven by perfectionism and fear of disappointing others. Ignoring her body's cues has dulled her awareness of hunger and fatigue. Her inner critic insists,* You're lazy if you slow down. *To cope, she keeps moving—working, exercising, planning. She turns to wine to quiet her mind and relax, but the relief is brief. By morning, guilt returns, and the cycle of stress and self-criticism continues.*

*Lauren learned to feel responsible for others while being a caregiver for her mother with MS. She pushes through fatigue and pain, and when her body signals exhaustion, she worries instead of resting. She copes by overanalyzing, withdrawing when burned out, burying herself in work, or stress eating—strategies that offer only brief relief and don't help her reset. She absorbs others' stress as her own. Carrying both her stress and everyone else's leaves her overwhelmed and trapped in cycles of fatigue and indecision.*

*Hailey interprets minor sensations as dangerous, repeatedly triggering her fight-or-flight response. Stress hormones amplify the sensations she fears, making her body feel even more alarmed. Because this cycle happens so often, her stress response rarely turns off, leading to fatigue, sleep issues, migraines, and increased pain sensitivity.*

*David has been under stress since his business partner's betrayal. He feels anxious about his business and his ability to support his family. Because he avoids conflict, the stress never fully subsides. His body shows the strain through tension, poor sleep, and fatigue. He avoids difficult emails at work and withdraws at home, coping through overeating and distraction. With low interoceptive awareness, he misses opportunities to regulate himself, and his coping strategies perpetuate the stress cycle.*

When we look at how people experience chronic stress and try to cope with it, we see how stress can hijack the body's internal signals, making it harder to understand what sensations mean or use them to regulate emotions. We also notice common patterns in how stress tends to show up. Stress responses often work to reduce exposure to anything that might add more strain; when someone's stress is already high, they naturally shift into behaviors that feel protective—even if those behaviors aren't healthy in the long run. For others, strong reactions emerge simply because their systems have become overloaded.

**Avoidance.** When people are stressed, they often try to limit their exposure to emotionally charged stimuli. They may shut down, withdraw from difficult conversations, or steer clear of conflict altogether. Some avoid social situations or relationships that might stir up uncomfortable emotions or require energy they don't have. Tasks that feel overwhelming get postponed or ignored. For a nervous system already under strain, avoiding anything that could add more stress feels logical—it's a way of protecting themselves from overload.

**Emotional suppression.** Others cope by pushing down or hiding their emotions. They may appear calm on the outside, but research shows this doesn't actually soothe the internal stress response. Philippe Goldin and colleagues note that emotion-related brain regions—especially the amygdala and insula—remain highly active even when feelings are suppressed. This often leads to increased physical stress, such as muscle tension or a racing heart. The emotion may seem less intense simply because the person is focused on keeping it contained.[5] If the amygdala is the brain's smoke alarm, emotional suppression is like turning off the alarm without putting out the fire.

**Busyness and overworking.** Staying busy allows people to keep their attention on tasks and responsibilities rather than on their internal experiences. Constant activity helps them avoid noticing bodily signals like fatigue, and emotions such as sadness or anger. By keeping their focus outward, they reduce the likelihood of being overwhelmed by what they might notice if they slowed down. Being "productive" can also create a sense of control when one's internal world feels uncomfortable or unpredictable.

**Hypervigilance.** In a state of chronic stress, the nervous system often stays on high alert. A person may remain attuned to signs of danger or threat, even when the actual risk is low. Depending on the individual, this heightened awareness may be directed toward their environment, their interactions with others, or their own internal sensations. They may be hypervigilant to potential safety threats, watchful for signs of rejection, or fearfully scanning their bodies for symptoms.

**Self-criticism and perfectionism.** For some people, internal sensations linked to mistakes or criticism feel especially unsafe—particularly if past errors were punished, shamed, or rejected. The nervous system shifts into protection mode and becomes sensitive to anything that might trigger those feelings again, such as errors, criticism, or perceived failure. Self-criticism develops as a way to prevent negative outcomes by harshly monitoring and correcting oneself before anyone else can. Perfectionism serves a similar purpose, aiming to avoid the shame or fear associated with mistakes. By striving to get everything right, the person is really trying to avoid the internal discomfort of feeling judged or inadequate.

**Emotional reactivity.** Chronic stress also makes people react quickly to anything that feels even slightly threatening. Minor frustrations or misunderstandings can trigger a fight-or-flight response. The nervous system, shaped by past stress, leans on strong emotions to take action, stay safe, or regain control. With time, this creates a cycle: Stress amplifies internal sensations, those sensations trigger emotional surges, and the surges reinforce the sense that the world is unsafe. Emotional reactivity is the body's way of protecting a person from additional stress—even though it often complicates relationships and makes self-regulation harder.

Though each person's story is unique, they illustrate a shared truth: When stress becomes chronic, the fight-or-flight system doesn't switch off. The body's signals—whether muted, distorted, or overwhelming—lose their reliability as guides. Without interoceptive balance, coping strategies often create more stress than they relieve, leaving individuals caught in loops of exhaustion, disconnection, and reactivity.

# 9

# Trauma Symptoms and Interoceptive Interruptions

It may be surprising to realize that trauma is a relatively recent concept in psychology. To put this in perspective, car alarms were already being installed in vehicles before post-traumatic stress disorder (PTSD) was officially recognized. Although car alarms appeared in the late 1960s and early 1970s, PTSD did not become an official diagnosis until 1980, when it was added to the *Diagnostic and Statistical Manual of Mental Disorders* (DSM-III).[1] Before then, traumatic experiences were often overlooked, and symptoms were dismissed as personal weakness rather than understood as a legitimate response to something overwhelming and frightening.

Our understanding has evolved dramatically since then. For decades, trauma was considered vague, shameful, or a sign of personal failing. Today, we recognize it as a serious condition with specific symptoms, shaped by both the body and the mind. We also know that trauma comes in many forms and that children are especially vulnerable, as it can profoundly impact their development. As discussed in the previous chapter, research shows trauma alters not only emotions and relationships but also the nervous system itself, including stress responses and our connection to interoceptive cues.

## Impacts of Cumulative Trauma

Alongside the growing awareness of trauma and its harmful effects, research has deepened our understanding of just how widespread it is. A landmark study published in 2015 reported that more than 70 percent of adults worldwide have experienced at least one traumatic event, and just over 30 percent have experienced four or more. In the United States, the numbers are even higher: The lifetime prevalence of any traumatic event is nearly 83 percent.[2] These statistics underscore the urgent need to recognize how profoundly trauma shapes people's everyday lives. The scale is staggering.

The Adverse Childhood Experiences (ACE) Study further highlights how common trauma is and how severe its long-term effects can be. Conducted in the 1990s by Vincent Felitti and colleagues, the study examined more than seventeen thousand American adults to explore the relationship between early adversity and adult health outcomes. Researchers identified ten types of adverse childhood experiences (ACEs), including abuse, neglect, and family challenges such as addiction, mental illness, violence, or incarceration. The study's key finding is that childhood adversity is both common and cumulative: The more ACEs a person experiences, the higher their risk for poor mental and physical health in adulthood. Higher ACE scores were strongly associated with depression, substance use, obesity, suicide attempts, and cancer. Only one-third of participants reported no ACEs, underscoring how widespread early adversity is and how powerfully it influences lifelong health.[3]

Importantly, the ACE framework does not capture all sources of trauma. Many people also experience medical trauma, car accidents, natural disasters, war, and social injustice. When these experiences are considered alongside ACEs, they provide a fuller picture of cumulative trauma and help explain why its effects often extend beyond what the ACE Study measures.

Bessel van der Kolk notes that "vast numbers of people who seek psychiatric care are, in fact, traumatized human beings."[4] His work has helped broaden our understanding of trauma as an experience that lives in both mind and body. This view is increasingly supported by research showing that interoceptive difficulties are common across mental health conditions and especially central to trauma and PTSD.[5]

In other words, unresolved trauma is more widespread than often acknowledged, and it shows up across a variety of mental health issues. Interoceptive disruptions are a key part of these difficulties, making it harder for people to feel safe and at home in their own bodies. These realities are the focus of the next two chapters, which unpack how trauma can create profound challenges to feeling secure and comfortable within oneself.

## Traumatic Stress and Interoceptive Disturbances

In the previous chapter, we looked at stress and its close connection to interoception. The stress response works much like a car alarm: It blares to warn of danger and quiets once the threat has passed. But with trauma, the alarm doesn't shut off. It keeps sounding even when there's no real danger. Everyday triggers—a loud noise, a smell, or even a passing thought—can set it off again. The body stays on high alert, bracing for threats that aren't there. Traumatic stress overloads the system, making it hard to tell real danger from false alarms.

Trauma occurs when an experience is so overwhelming or threatening that it disrupts a person's sense of safety, stability, or ability to cope. Events such as assault, abuse, or serious accidents can leave survivors feeling fear, helplessness, or horror. Unlike everyday stress, recovery often takes far longer. People may experience nightmares, flashbacks, or intense emotions that don't fade, leaving the body and brain stuck in fight-or-flight mode. For many, this chronic hyperarousal disrupts sleep, mood, and memory, while physical symptoms and intrusive memories keep the body's alarm system activated. Just as chronic stress interferes with awareness of bodily signals, traumatic stress does so in even more profound ways.

People who have experienced trauma often misinterpret or fear their own bodily sensations, making regulation and recovery more challenging. Trauma can alter how a person perceives and interprets what's happening in their body and environment, causing even ordinary sensations to feel confusing or frightening. The nervous system may become overly sensitive, leading to overwhelm and a constant sense of being on edge. For others, trauma has the opposite effect, creating numbness or diminished sensitivity, including difficulty feeling pain.[6] In both cases, the body is adapting in ways meant to protect the person, but these changes can make everyday sensations feel either too intense or too distant. These extremes—feeling too much or too little—are hallmark patterns in how trauma reshapes the body's sensory experience.

## Hyperarousal and Hypoarousal

The stress response is normally adaptive and temporary—a survival mechanism that turns off once the danger has passed. But with significant trauma, especially when it occurs repeatedly or early in life, this system can become dysregulated. Instead of returning to a more regulated baseline, the stress response stays elevated, driving many symptoms of PTSD. Survivors often perceive bodily sensations differently, caught between two disrupted states that clinicians describe as *hyperarousal* and *hypoarousal.*

Hyperarousal is the "too much" side: The body remains on high alert, with anxiety, irritability, anger, muscle tension, trembling, or exaggerated startle responses. These overwhelming sensations make it difficult to regulate emotions or interpret internal cues, as if the alarm never turns off. Hypoarousal is the "too little" side: The nervous system shuts down, leading to disconnection, numbness, and a dulled awareness of bodily signals. In both cases, trauma affects the natural link between body and mind.

Research suggests that roughly 70 percent of people with PTSD experience predominantly hyperarousal symptoms, while about 30 percent experience hypoarousal.[7] Yet these numbers only tell part of the story. Many trauma survivors shift rapidly between the two states rather than remaining in one. The common thread is a struggle to feel safe and at ease in the body. Trauma profoundly disrupts the mind–body connection, often leaving people less aware of—or less able to trust—their inner experiences. Understanding trauma in this way highlights just how deeply it reshapes a person's relationship with themselves.

## Hyperarousal Symptoms of Trauma

Many of the symptoms related to hyperarousal can seem overwhelming or excessive. And many of them involved physical sensations.

### *Nervous System Arousal*

Trauma can keep the nervous system locked in a state of heightened arousal, marked by hypervigilance, exaggerated startle responses, sensitivity to noise or light, sleep disturbance, and intrusive reminders of the past. These effects are often amplified by childhood trauma, since early experiences influence how the stress system develops. As a result, even ordinary situations may feel threatening, and emotional reactions may become disproportionate to the circumstances.

Traumatic experiences trigger an extreme stress response, resulting in intense physical sensations, such as a rapid heartbeat or muscle tension. These bodily cues often become linked with traumatic memories, reinforcing hyperarousal, heightened reactivity, and reexperiencing symptoms. In time, trauma interferes with the nervous system's capacity for self-regulation, leading to long-term emotional and physical challenges.

*In addition to early attachment wounds from emotionally absent parents, Ava was sexually assaulted by her boyfriend in high school. Although she appeared to move on afterward, the impact remains evident in her nervous system. She is now hypervigilant in social situations, highly sensitive to rejection and criticism, and has experienced ongoing sleep difficulties since the assault.*

*Jason grew up with an abusive, alcoholic father, leaving his body constantly on alert. He reacts with frustration to small things, like a supervisor's correction, a partner's question, or a coworker's joke. Calmness feels unfamiliar to him, while vigilance, irritability, and anger are his usual responses.*

## *Physical Symptoms*

When the stress response stays activated, it contributes to the challenging physical symptoms that occur when the body is under pressure. We looked at these in the previous chapter on stress. The symptoms include muscle tension, body aches, and headaches, as stress causes muscles to tense up as part of the fight-or-flight response. When stress remains, the tension persists. Gastrointestinal discomfort is also common for those with unresolved trauma, since it disrupts digestive processes and contributes to nausea, heartburn, bloating, constipation, or diarrhea.

## *Unmanageable Emotions*

Hyperarousal doesn't just keep the body on edge; it also unleashes powerful emotions like anger, fear, shame, and irritability. These feelings are inseparable from bodily sensations: a racing heart, a tight chest, or a sinking feeling in the stomach. For trauma survivors, such signals often feel overwhelming or frightening, fueling a cycle in which sensations and emotions amplify each other. As Van der Kolk explains, trauma makes it hard to use emotions as cues; instead of noticing a trigger and making sense of it, people with PTSD often jump straight from trigger to reaction, as if the fight-or-flight switch is stuck *on*.[8]

*Catherine feels deep shame from her mother's harsh criticism. As a child, making mistakes made her feel she wasn't good enough, and as an adult, even small errors still trigger that same sense of unworthiness. She fears disappointing others, which pushes her to overperform. When she tries to rest or set boundaries, she feels guilty. Her nervous system remains on high alert, and she uses constant busyness to manage her anxiety. Instead of expressing anger, Catherine turns it inward through self-criticism.*

*Ava carries intense emotions from being assaulted by someone she trusted. The experience left her confused and self-blaming, and because it was never processed, shame became tied to her body image. Even small criticisms now trigger that shame, leading to anger or frantic attempts to fix her appearance. The betrayal also left her mistrustful and hypervigilant in relationships. When parents set limits or partners disappoint her, the old wound resurfaces, and her emotions spill out as defensiveness, tears, or rage.*

*Early abuse by his alcoholic father left Jason carrying deep fear and shame. As a child, fear kept him on edge, while shame grew from feeling powerless and unworthy. Because these emotions felt unsafe to express, he learned to bury them and replace vulnerability with anger. As an adult, anger dominates his emotional world. When he feels stressed or criticized, the old fear and shame surface but are experienced as rage, often leading to explosive reactions.*

### *Intrusive Symptoms*

Intrusive symptoms such as flashbacks, nightmares, and unwanted thoughts about trauma add additional layers to interoceptive disturbances. Instead of staying in the past, traumatic memories often intrude into the present, not as a clear story but as fragments: disturbing images, overwhelming body sensations, or waves of intense emotion. A person might suddenly feel their heart racing, their chest tightening, or terror washing over them as if the trauma were happening again. These intrusions keep the nervous system ready and braced for danger. In this way, intrusive symptoms do more than remind someone of what happened—they actively sustain the cycle of hyperarousal, preventing the body and mind from relaxing.

*Catherine's experience of emotional abuse, high pressure, and conditional love has led to intrusive symptoms that appear subtly but still disrupt her daily life. She repeatedly has unwanted memories of her mother's harsh words. She replays moments when she was humiliated or berated, especially after small mistakes. Fear and shame are reinforced as she has internalized her mother's critical voice: "Don't be lazy," "You didn't try hard enough." Catherine also notices how tense she feels when she anticipates disapproval or feedback from a colleague or boss.*

*Because Ava has pushed her traumatic experiences out of her awareness, she doesn't always recognize that her intrusive symptoms are connected to the assault. Her sleep is restless and filled with unsettling dreams, and she often scrolls on her phone late into the night to avoid going to bed. Waves of shame, fear, or disgust can hit her suddenly, especially when she feels criticized, rejected, or emotionally exposed. She also has sudden flashbacks, particularly during intimate moments.*

*At times, her body reacts even without clear memories—a racing heart, nausea, or tight muscles that make her feel as though she's reliving the experience all over again.*

## Coping Behaviors

People who have experienced overwhelming events often develop patterns of avoidance or distraction to cope with the intense emotions and distressing symptoms that follow. Since overwhelming experiences produce intense sensations, many survivors naturally turn to behaviors that temporarily dull, soothe, or redirect those feelings. These can include substance use, disordered eating, high-risk activities, aggression, or compulsive behaviors like gambling or excessive use of digital media.

Research also shows that exposure to traumatic events can lead to chronic avoidance. These strategies often seem helpful initially because they reduce trauma-related tension or intrusive emotional states. However, over time, they can become ingrained habits that hinder emotional processing and keep individuals disconnected from their internal experiences. Trauma experts note that individuals with trauma histories may resort to substances or other means of tension reduction to dampen the distress linked to traumatic events or memories.[9] Gabor Maté similarly emphasizes that many avoidance patterns arise as attempts to escape the inner distress created by trauma, explaining that "hurt is at the centre of all addictive behaviors."[10] From this perspective, these behaviors—whether substance-related or not—are less about seeking pleasure and more about easing the distress that feels too overwhelming to face directly.

*When Catherine feels shame or fears judgment, she copes by overworking and overfunctioning. She takes extra shifts and plans family events to drown out painful emotions and prove her worth. She says yes to almost everything to avoid criticism. Her perfectionism drives her to overprepare and set impossible standards, offering brief control but constant pressure. She suppresses her body's signals, pushing through hunger, pain, and exhaustion rather than slowing down. By day's end, she turns to wine to quiet her inner critic, but the relief is temporary, and guilt pulls her back into the cycle.*

*Ava relies on coping strategies that bring brief relief but keep her stuck in the long run. When shame or fear shows up, she rigidly controls her body—restricting food, overexercising, or obsessing over her appearance. She spends hours perfecting her online image and endlessly scrolling through social media. While scrolling distracts her, it also fuels comparison and stress. She seeks external validation to soothe herself, depending on likes, comments, and gifts from partners to quiet her insecurities. She also avoids discomfort by retreating into her online world. These patterns keep her in survival mode, numbing her triggers without truly resolving them.*

*When Jason feels overwhelmed by trauma triggers like criticism or conflict, he turns to behaviors that numb, avoid, or discharge emotions rather than regulate them. Alcohol is his primary coping strategy, easing tension briefly before leaving him more irritable and primed to explode. He also suppresses emotions—pushing sadness, fear, and vulnerability out of awareness. Jason also relies on impulsive actions, such as picking fights, storming out, or taking risks at work, to release tension. These strategies offer quick relief but reinforce hyperarousal and keep him stuck in survival mode.*

## Hypoarousal Symptoms of Trauma

Just as some trauma symptoms feel overwhelming or too much, others fall on the opposite end of the spectrum. Hypoarousal occurs when the nervous system shuts down instead of remaining on high alert, shifting into a freeze or collapse response. When experiences feel too intense to process, the body protects itself by numbing, slowing down, or disconnecting from feelings and sensations. Eventually, this survival strategy can become a lasting pattern, manifesting as fatigue, emotional numbness, dissociation, or a sense of detachment from one's body or surroundings. In essence, hypoarousal is the nervous system's attempt to cope with overwhelm by shutting down.

### *Nervous System Arousal*

When looking at the nervous system impacts, hypoarousal often feels like a disconnection between body and mind. Breathing may become shallow, muscles heavy, and energy depleted, creating sensations of lethargy or collapse. Dissociation can emerge, leaving a person feeling spacey, detached from the body, or as if observing themselves from the outside. Basic internal cues—such as hunger, pain, or touch—may be dulled or absent, reinforcing a pervasive sense of numbness. This shutdown not only distances individuals from their bodily experience but also creates a profound sense of separation from the world around them. Neuroimaging studies support this, showing reduced activation in the insula, a brain region central to interoceptive awareness.[11] This helps explain why hypoarousal so often leaves people feeling profoundly disconnected from themselves.

*Roland often appears flat and emotionally distant, which is his version of hypoarousal. His body remains subdued and underresponsive, leaving him disconnected from his own stress signals and chances for genuine relational connection.*

*David often exhibits hypoarousal symptoms, his body and mind defaulting to numbness and withdrawal. He wakes up already exhausted, with little motivation to get through his day, and often ends up on the couch instead of engaging with his family.*

## Emotions

In hypoarousal, emotions often seem muted because the person isn't fully present in their body. When bodily sensations are dulled or absent, the emotional experiences that normally arise from those sensations are also dampened. This can appear as numbness, avoidance, or a sense of emotional disconnection, where feelings seem distant or flat. Pleasure and joy are absent, while despair, hopelessness, helplessness, and depression can take over. It's not that the emotions are gone, but without the body's signals to guide them, they become dulled, leaving the person feeling cut off from themselves and others.

*For Roland, hypoarousal shows up in how little he experiences emotionally. He often feels "nothing," reflecting a nervous system that stays shut down. His inner world is muted—he rarely laughs, shows excitement, or recognizes sadness, anger, or joy. Curiosity and playfulness are limited. When his wife seeks connection, he feels no desire for closeness. When family members are frustrated with him, it hardly registers.*

*David's emotions have become quiet, buried under numbness and withdrawal. He feels flat or empty, with joy out of reach and sadness dulled into heaviness. This shutdown stems from unresolved grief over losing his father at fourteen and from the impact of his mother's depression, which formed an early pattern of emotional detachment that returns when life feels overwhelming. This numbed state reinforces his belief that he's failing his family and deepens the cycle of disconnection and despair.*

## Behavioral Patterns

When someone is stuck in hypoarousal, the effects extend beyond body and emotion into daily life. People may withdraw from social interactions, isolate themselves, or avoid responsibilities because being present feels overwhelming. Avoidance becomes a way of existing: relationships, self-care, and even basic needs like hunger can fade into the background. In time, these patterns of withdrawal and restriction deepen the sense of disconnection.

With interoceptive signals already dulled in hypoarousal, such behaviors make it even harder to recognize what the body needs, leaving a person more detached from themselves and the world around them. As Peter Levine observes, shutting down distressing feelings also shuts down the capacity to notice subtle signals of comfort or satisfaction. In turn, pleasure itself becomes inaccessible: "You can't have it both ways; when feelings of dread are held at bay, so are the feelings of joy."[12]

*Roland distances himself from his emotions by overworking and intellectualizing, choosing to explain things through logic or facts. He also dismisses health concerns and relational complaints as "overreacting," protecting himself from discomfort but missing important cues.*

*David withdraws and avoids, pulling back from his wife and sons, retreating to the couch, and sidestepping conflict at home and work. He dismisses responsibilities with "It doesn't matter anyway" and downplays his feelings as being "just tired." He's disengaged from activities he once enjoyed and now numbs himself with food and scrolling on his phone. These habits briefly dull emotional pain but keep him disconnected and stuck in hypoarousal.*

## Experiencing Both Hyper- and Hypoarousal

Although people often show a pattern of either hyperarousal or hypoarousal, those who have experienced trauma frequently shift between hyperarousal, where sensations become overwhelming and chaotic, and hypoarousal, where signals are dulled or absent. They can encounter both extremes, each of which erodes interoceptive awareness.

*While Jason's life is dominated by hyperarousal symptoms, he does slip into hypoarousal through his patterns of suppressing emotions, numbing with alcohol, and disconnection from his bodily cues.*

*Catherine is also highly activated and in hyperarousal often. She uses alcohol to give herself permission to slow down and numb out.*

*David experiences both but leans toward hypoarousal. We can see this in his general state of fatigue and low energy, but he also has periods*

***of intense anxiety and worry. One moment, his mind is racing and his body feels tense; the next, he's collapsed on the couch.***

As Peter Levine observes, traumatized people are "trapped between feeling too much or too little." Unable to trust their sensations, they lose their way.[13] In this sense, a loss of sensation becomes a loss of self. Whether the nervous system is stuck in "too much" or "too little" activation, trauma disrupts the mind–body connection, turning internal signals into sources of fear or emptiness instead of guidance. Both states significantly impair interoception and cause a pervasive lack of safety and comfort within one's own body—an experience that is painfully common among those who have lived through trauma.

Viewing these disruptions through the lens of interoception explains why survivors often feel unsafe inside their bodies and why healing involves restoring a balanced, trustworthy connection to inner experience. The next chapter will focus on how trauma affects the aspects of interoception measured by the MAIA.

# 10

# Trauma and the Disrupted Sense of Self

In college, my friends and I often played hide-and-seek in one of the campus buildings, and during one game, several of us hid in a large dressing room with no ambient light. When the others left, I wasn't quick enough to follow and suddenly found myself alone in absolute darkness, unsure where the door was. At first, I tried to rely on touch, tracing the walls to orient myself. But then I unexpectedly bumped into a friend I didn't know was there. A prankster, he spun me around until I lost all sense of direction. In the pitch-black room, I became completely disoriented—unable to rely on sight and cut off from the cues that usually help us figure things out. The experience was brief and harmless, but it left me with a striking memory of what it feels like to lose trust in your own internal signals.

Just as I needed help to find my way out, trauma can leave people disoriented within themselves, struggling to navigate their own bodily signals without guidance. The research is clear: Traumatic experiences can leave survivors feeling unable to make sense of the signals their bodies are sending. This disruption of interoception often creates a profound sense of disorientation and uncertainty about one's inner world.

## Trauma, Interoception, and the Loss of Self

Peter Levine is a leading expert in body-oriented approaches to trauma and the developer of Somatic Experiencing, a method that helps people resolve trauma by focusing on the body's responses to overwhelming experiences. He writes: "Unable to trust their sensations, traumatized people can lose their way. They don't 'feel like themselves' anymore; loss of sensation equals a loss of a sense of self."[1]

What happens when people lose this sense of self? As a trauma therapist, I've worked with many clients who struggle to make sense of their thoughts, feelings, behaviors, and relationship patterns. They are often bewildered by their own reactions. A common thread running through these struggles is disrupted interoception. When trauma distorts the ability to notice and trust internal cues, people may feel anxious without knowing why, be overwhelmed by emotions they cannot regulate, self-medicate unidentified distress, or misjudge their needs in relationships. Put simply, many of the challenges we see in therapy—whether anxiety, addiction, eating disorders, or relational turmoil—stem from the disorientation and disconnection that begin in the body. And when survivors have difficulty accurately identifying and interpreting their bodily sensations, managing the rest of their trauma symptoms becomes far more challenging.

In the previous chapter, we looked at trauma and how it can manifest as physical, emotional, and behavioral symptoms in people who have experienced it. Now, we'll use the MAIA to explore how trauma and its symptoms can interfere with interoceptive processes—and why this disruption is so destabilizing to a person's sense of self. You may find it helpful to revisit the earlier chapter to see how the case studies involving hyperarousal and hypoarousal map onto different MAIA criteria.

Before we examine how trauma affects interoceptive awareness through the lens of the MAIA domains, it's important to remember that not all interoceptive challenges stem from trauma. As we've seen throughout the book, stressful life experiences, health conditions, and attachment patterns can also shape how people perceive and respond to bodily cues. With this in mind, we can now look at how trauma specifically alters interoception.

### *1. Noticing: Awareness of Physical Sensations*

As we learned earlier, noticing interoceptive cues means paying attention to what's happening inside the body—breathing, tension, warmth, or a racing heart—without immediately trying to fix or judge these sensations. This awareness can foster self-understanding since bodily signals carry essential information about needs and states. However, being a good noticer of bodily sensations is only helpful when paired with the ability to regulate those sensations and manage worry. Trauma complicates this process.

Some trauma survivors experience little connection to their bodily sensations—they show the hypoarousal pattern in noticing internal cues. But others become more sensitive to their body signals, a form of hyperarousal. Heightened awareness of cues like a racing heart or muscle tremors can make these sensations feel threatening, fueling a vicious cycle; fear of the signals amplifies the stress response, which in turn worsens symptoms. For these survivors, increased bodily awareness becomes more of a burden than a benefit. Beyond anxiety and hypervigilance, it may appear as health anxiety or chronic pain conditions such as IBS and fibromyalgia, with heightened sensitivity only deepening their suffering.

As Van der Kolk observes in *The Body Keeps the Score*: "The more [traumatized] people try to push away and ignore internal warning signs, the more likely they are to take over and leave them bewildered, confused, and ashamed. People who cannot comfortably notice what is going on inside become vulnerable to respond to any sensory shift either by shutting down or by going into a panic."[2]

## *2. Not-Distracting: Tendency Not to Ignore or Distract from Uncomfortable Sensations*

Not distracting from body signals means being willing to notice discomfort instead of numbing it with food, alcohol, constant busyness, or other distractions like social media. While avoidance might bring temporary relief, it prevents people from recognizing what they truly need. Those who struggle in this area often suppress or push away uncomfortable sensations, which only adds stress and delays healing. In contrast, being able to sit with discomfort—without necessarily liking it—reflects stronger self-awareness and a healthier, more balanced relationship with the body.

Of course, this is easier said than done. Trauma symptoms can be incredibly hard to sit with. Hyperarousal brings hypervigilance, startling easily, muscle tension, nightmares, intrusive thoughts, and overwhelming emotions. Hypoarousal, on the other hand, can feel like disconnection—numbness, detachment from self or others, and a flat, joyless existence. Given how painful both ends of the spectrum are, it's understandable that survivors look for ways to escape.

When I worked at an addiction treatment center, I saw firsthand that people don't develop addictions by accident—they are almost always self-medicating something. The link between trauma and addiction is undeniable. Trauma produces unbearable symptoms, many of which are rooted in overwhelming bodily sensations. Addiction and other forms of distraction are often a desperate attempt to quiet those signals.

### 3. Not-Worrying: Tendency Not to Worry About Unpleasant Sensations or Respond with Distress

This aspect of interoceptive awareness reflects how much people worry about their bodily sensations. Staying calm during discomfort—such as pain, tension, or fatigue—helps prevent anxious spirals. People with higher scores in this area can notice unpleasant sensations and respond in healthier, more adaptive ways without becoming overwhelmed. In contrast, excessive worry fuels overthinking and catastrophic thoughts, creating a vicious cycle of distress. A more helpful approach is to observe the body's signals with curiosity rather than fear, which fosters a stronger and healthier mind–body connection.

Worrying about bodily sensations often triggers a negative feedback loop: an interoceptive cue is interpreted as a warning that something is wrong, which intensifies the sensation and leads to further worry. Over time, even normal bodily signals—such as muscle tension, digestive activity, or fatigue—can become amplified and perceived as threatening. This process, known as *somatic amplification*, makes everyday sensations more challenging to ignore and more distressing than they need to be.

People with a history of trauma are especially vulnerable to this cycle. A large meta-analysis found they were nearly three times more likely to develop functional somatic disorders—conditions in which people experience real and debilitating symptoms, such as pain, exhaustion, or digestive difficulties, despite no clear medical explanation.[3] These disorders arise when the body's alarm system becomes overly sensitive, causing normal signals to feel stronger, more uncomfortable, and less tolerable. Examples include IBS, fibromyalgia, and chronic fatigue syndrome. The symptoms are genuine and distressing, but they stem from how the brain and body process signals rather than from ongoing tissue damage. Trauma can prime this system to remain on high alert, making worry about bodily discomfort more likely to lead to chronic, disabling symptoms.

### 4. Attention Regulation: Ability to Regulate Attention to Bodily Sensations

This skill involves mindfully noticing bodily sensations—such as heartbeat, breath, or muscle tension—while gently refocusing the mind when it wanders. The goal is balance: staying present without becoming overwhelmed or disconnected. Developing this capacity helps people recognize emotions, physical needs, and sources of discomfort.

Trauma can profoundly disrupt a person's sense of identity, affecting both how they think about themselves and how they physically experience their body. People with PTSD often describe feeling disconnected, emotionally numb, or unfamiliar to themselves. Ruth Lanius has conducted extensive research connecting these experiences to brain processes. The brain system most involved in creating our sense of self is the default mode network (DMN), a group of brain regions active when we reflect on ourselves or recall personal memories. In healthy individuals, the DMN operates smoothly during rest, helping maintain a stable, continuous sense of identity. For those with PTSD, this network becomes less connected and less coordinated. The more disrupted it is, the more severe the person's trauma symptoms tend to be.[4]

Through the lens of the MAIA, this disruption often shows up as difficulty sustaining attention to inner experience. Instead of supporting healthy reflection, the DMN can get stuck in trauma-based identities tied to overwhelming sensations. Fragmented memory further pulls attention away from the present. Some survivors feel flooded by their bodies, while others go numb and disconnect—both patterns undermine the ability to pay attention to bodily experiences. Trauma triggers can also hijack the DMN, making it harder to return to calming or neutral sensations. Put simply, when trauma disrupts the DMN, it weakens our capacity to anchor in the body and stay present.

## *5. Emotional Awareness: Ability to Recognize the Connection Between Bodily Sensations and Emotions*

Emotional awareness is the ability to notice how feelings show up in the body, such as linking muscle tension with stress, a racing heart with fear, or butterflies with excitement. Tuning into these signals helps us distinguish between emotions, understand ourselves better, and manage our feelings in healthier ways. When awareness is low, coping becomes harder; when it's strong, it supports resilience, connection, and stability. Trauma survivors often struggle in this area. Some rely on dissociation or disconnection, which numbs emotional signals. Others live with hyperarousal that floods the nervous system and blurs the line between physical and emotional states. Trauma can also bring waves of intense, overwhelming emotions that feel so unsafe that survivors shut down or avoid them altogether.

One common pattern of reduced emotional awareness is *alexithymia*—difficulty identifying and expressing emotions. Research shows it is especially prevalent among people with PTSD, who score higher on alexithymia than trauma-exposed individuals without PTSD. Not only is it more common, but it is also tied to more severe PTSD symptoms, suggesting that challenges with emotional awareness may intensify trauma's impact.[5] Those with alexithymia often confuse emotions with basic bodily states, such as hunger or fatigue, making regulation difficult. The condition also disrupts empathy, decision-making, and relationships, as what people say they feel often doesn't match their body's signals.[6] For example, someone might insist they aren't angry even while their heart races and their muscles are tight. This mismatch makes it harder to convey emotions clearly.

Alexithymia often develops in childhood, especially when caregivers fail to express or respond to emotions in healthy ways. Growing up with distant or inconsistent caregivers can make it difficult to recognize and describe one's own feelings later in life. This illustrates how both trauma and early emotional experiences influence our ability to connect with our emotions.[7] Consider Roland and his challenges with emotional awareness, relational disconnection, and his reduced ability to interpret bodily cues. He meets the criteria for alexithymia, including his history of childhood attachment trauma and his pattern of avoidant attachment.

Emotional awareness is a foundational skill that precedes emotional regulation. Before we can manage our feelings in healthy ways, we first need to notice, accept, and accurately label them. Without that foundation, regulation strategies have little to build on. This is why people with trauma histories, especially those with alexithymia, often struggle to regulate their emotions. If it's difficult to recognize and name what they're feeling in the first place, it's understandable that managing those emotions becomes even harder.

### *6. Self-Regulation: Ability to Regulate Distress Through Attention to Bodily Sensations*

Self-regulation is the ability to notice bodily signals—like tension or a racing heart—and respond with healthy strategies. People with strong self-regulation recognize early stress cues and use techniques such as deep breathing or relaxation to stay calm. Those with weaker skills may overlook these signals, react impulsively, and struggle to manage stress.

Difficulties with self-regulation often overlap with other interoceptive challenges: over- or undernoticing bodily cues, becoming easily distracted, worrying excessively about sensations, struggling to use the body as a calming resource, or lacking emotional awareness. Because emotion regulation is a key component of self-regulation, unhelpful strategies such as avoidance or self-criticism tend to intensify distress.

Within the MAIA framework, attention regulation and self-regulation are closely related but distinct concepts. Attention regulation is the ability to sustain focus on bodily sensations without distraction. Self-regulation is the next step—using that awareness to calm distress and restore balance. Trauma often disrupts both, making body signals feel unsafe and undermining the body's role as a grounding resource.

When self-regulation breaks down, everyday life becomes more complicated to manage. Minor stressors can escalate into anger, tears, or intense anxiety. Coping often involves avoidance, withdrawal, or numbing through food, substances, or endless scrolling. Others may turn to risky behaviors—such as self-harm, reckless spending, or unsafe sex—that bring temporary relief but deepen dysregulation. At its core, poor self-regulation makes it difficult to regain balance after stress, leaving the body feeling unsafe rather than grounded.

### *7. Body Listening: Ability to Actively Listen to the Body for Insight or Guidance*

As a reminder, body listening is the practice of tuning into inner signals—like fatigue, emotions, or subtle bodily cues—and using them to guide self-care and decision-making. It's not just about noticing sensations but also interpreting them in supportive ways, such as resting when tired or acknowledging feelings as they arise. People who are skilled in body listening see these signals as valuable information, which builds self-awareness and encourages healthier responses to stress, emotions, and physical needs. Those who struggle with this skill often miss important signs about their health and well-being.

Even before I learned about the MAIA, I saw how difficult body listening can be for trauma survivors. Some of my clients were confused by the invitation to notice their bodies; others avoided it by focusing on their thoughts; and some were even irritated by the opportunity to be curious about their internal sensations. Individuals with PTSD or trauma histories often score low on the body listening domain, meaning they rarely consult their bodies when trying to understand emotions or make decisions. They may dismiss bodily cues as irrelevant or confusing, struggle to use somatic awareness for self-regulation, and instead rely on avoidance or external signals. Many describe difficulty connecting body states to emotions, saying things like, "I don't know what my body is telling me."

This pattern often reflects dissociation, numbing, or deliberate avoidance of interoceptive signals. For some, bodily sensations trigger distressing memories or hyperarousal, leading them to disconnect from their physical experience. As a result, emotions can feel confusing, overwhelming, or as though they appear out of nowhere. Instead of curiosity, survivors may respond to bodily sensations with fear or avoidance. Unfortunately, when body listening is impaired, so is the ability to care for the body in effective and compassionate ways.

### *8. Trusting: Experience of One's Body as Safe and Trustworthy*

Trusting bodily sensations means seeing the body as a safe, reliable source of information. When we feel secure in our bodies, we can approach discomfort with curiosity and use internal signals to guide self-care. Low body trust, by contrast, creates disconnection and makes healthy choices harder.

Trauma often disrupts this sense of safety. Because traumatic experiences often involve the body being threatened or violated, survivors may lose confidence in what their bodies are telling them. For someone with PTSD, normal sensations—like a racing heart or tight chest—can feel dangerous, interpreted as signs of threat. In time, the body comes to feel untrustworthy, leading many survivors to tune out or numb their sensations. As Bessel van der Kolk notes, "traumatized people chronically feel unsafe in their bodies," and this deep mistrust drives many of the struggles they face.[8]

This disconnection shows up in daily life. Survivors may avoid noticing physical sensations or slip into dissociation. Hyperarousal—constantly feeling on edge, jumpy, or scanning for danger—only reinforces the belief that bodily signals can't be trusted. Everyday needs like hunger, fatigue, or pain are often ignored because tuning in feels unsafe. Without reliable cues, even basic self-care, such as eating, resting, or slowing down, becomes difficult. And since emotions are rooted in bodily sensations, distrusting the body also undermines emotional regulation, leaving survivors vulnerable to sudden overwhelm or shutdown. In this way, trauma transforms the body from a trusted ally into something that feels unsafe.

The loss of body trust also affects relationships, particularly in recognizing danger signals. Normally, the body warns us through gut feelings, tension, or a pounding heart. But trauma can dull or distort these cues. What is unsafe can come to feel familiar or acceptable, while safety feels strange or unsettling. Survivors may numb fear or discomfort, endure harmful behaviors longer, or second-guess their instincts—telling themselves they're overreacting even when their body signals danger. This erosion of body trust weakens the internal warning system, making it harder to leave—or easier to return to—abusive relationships.

## Trauma and Interoceptive Disruptions

Unresolved trauma often changes how people experience their own bodies. Signals that would normally guide rest, safety, or self-care can instead feel confusing, overwhelming, or difficult to trust. Some people begin to tune out or numb bodily sensations, while others become intensely aware of them—especially when those sensations signal distress. Trauma rarely alters body awareness in just one way. Instead, it shifts the balance. Sensations may become more noticeable yet harder to interpret, regulate, or rely on. Over time, the body can start to feel less like a steady guide and more like the first place where distress shows up.

When this happens, people may begin to avoid their internal cues altogether. If paying attention to the body brings discomfort rather than relief, it makes it harder to link sensations with emotions or respond to them in supportive ways. Instead of offering guidance and regulation, the body may seem unpredictable or untrustworthy. This disconnection can ripple outward, affecting emotional steadiness, resilience, relationships, and overall well-being.

Yet interoception also offers a path forward. With support and practice, individuals can learn to notice their body's signals with curiosity rather than fear, gradually rebuilding a sense of safety and trust within themselves. As internal cues become easier to tolerate and understand, they can shift from being sources of distress to sources of guidance. Cultivating this mind–body connection strengthens resilience and healing, helping restore a more grounded and integrated sense of self.

# Part Three

# CHALLENGES WITH INTEROCEPTION

# 11

# Common Threads, Synergistic Impacts, and Unintended Consequences

We have explored interoception as a key process in how the body functions, how emotions are experienced and regulated, and how mental health is shaped. We've seen how disruptions in interoception can stem from trauma, early attachment experiences, ongoing stress, and unhelpful thought patterns. These factors do not occur in isolation; they interact and influence one another. For instance, anxious thoughts can heighten bodily sensations, chronic stress can reinforce a sense of constant threat, and early relational experiences can make it harder to notice or respond to internal signals.

Interoception is not just an abstract idea; it directly affects how people feel, cope, and act in everyday life. When multiple interoceptive disruptions occur, their combined effects can begin to resemble specific mental or physical health conditions. Recognizing this helps move beyond a one-size-fits-all approach to mental health challenges. It encourages curiosity about how interoceptive disruptions accumulate and contribute to different conditions, and it helps us see how interoceptive awareness can be reshaped to enhance mental and physical well-being.

Unintended consequences remind us that even well-meaning actions can lead to unexpected results. When antibiotics first appeared, they were life-saving drugs that revolutionized medicine by curing bacterial infections. However, over time, their excessive use has caused serious side effects: Many bacteria have evolved into superbugs resistant to multiple antibiotics. Sometimes, actions aimed at solving one problem can unintentionally create much larger issues.

## Where's the Well-Being?

When we step back and look at the current state of global health and mental health, the picture is alarming. Here's what the numbers reveal about the scale of the struggles many people are facing:

**Mental health and substance use.** According to the World Health Organization (WHO), as of 2025, nearly one in seven people worldwide lives with a mental health disorder. Anxiety and depression are among the most common issues: About 4.4 percent of the global population currently experiences an anxiety disorder, while 4 percent experiences depression.[1] In the United States, the statistics are even more concerning. In 2024, nearly one in four adults—roughly sixty-one million people—had a mental health condition, including more than fourteen million with a serious mental illness that significantly impacts daily functioning.[2]

Substance use problems remain widespread as well. A 2024 WHO report estimates that nearly half a billion people worldwide are affected by substance use disorders, and treatment remains unavailable or unaffordable for many who need it most.[3]

**Problematic technology use.** Mood-altering behaviors extend beyond using substances. Many adults struggle with the overuse of technology and its negative effects on well-being and relationships. One 2023 review found that 37 to 66 percent of university students in several Asian and Middle Eastern countries experience problematic smartphone use. Social media, gaming, and pornography are key drivers, with young adults spending several hours a day on digital platforms and frequently reporting higher anxiety, depression, and sleep disturbances associated with heavy use.[4]

**Self-harm and suicidality.** Few issues reveal the extent of human suffering more starkly than suicide and self-harm. Suicide remains among the leading causes of death worldwide.[5] In the United States alone, over fourteen million adults report serious thoughts of suicide each year.[6]

Globally, self-harm among youth is widespread. Research across seventeen countries shows that nearly 18 percent of young people aged ten through nineteen have engaged in nonsuicidal self-injury (NSSI). Rates are higher among girls and young women (about 21 percent) than among boys and young men (nearly 14 percent).[7] These numbers represent millions of adolescents who use self-harm to cope with overwhelming internal distress.

**Chronic health issues.** An estimated 129 million people in the United States live with at least one chronic disease, including diabetes, heart disease, and cancer. Many of these conditions are linked to preventable risk factors such as smoking, poor nutrition, obesity, heavy alcohol use, and physical inactivity.[8] Most health-care spending in the United States is directed toward the long-term management and treatment of chronic diseases and mental health conditions.

**Interpersonal challenges and loneliness.** Growing disconnection, polarization, and rising aggression indicate that our relationships are under increasing strain. Incidents of public hostility reveal a decline in everyday civility, while increases in hate incidents and discrimination point to widening social and cultural divides. The pervasive influence of technology compounds these issues, contributing to an alarming trend toward reduced empathy and more superficial engagement on social media platforms.

Loneliness has become widespread as well: In 2022, about 24 percent of the global population reported feeling "very" or "fairly" lonely.[9] The health impact is significant—disconnection from others raises the risk of depression, anxiety, cardiovascular disease, and early death.

## Interoceptive Disruptions as a Common Thread

What if many human struggles could be better understood by examining shared roots in how we sense and interpret our bodies? Often, seemingly different symptoms arise from a single underlying issue. For example, a nutrient-deficient diet may show up as anemia, fatigue, brain fog, brittle nails, or bleeding gums—distinct problems stemming from the same cause.

In mental health research, such shared roots are known as *transdiagnostic mechanisms*. Martina Saltafossi and her colleagues describe altered interoception as one such mechanism, referring to it as a "common thread" linking mood and anxiety disorders.[10] While diagnostic systems such as the DSM separate conditions like depression, anxiety, and PTSD, growing evidence suggests that these disorders may share underlying interoceptive disruptions.

Many of these difficulties involve the brain's interoceptive network, particularly the insula, which processes bodily sensations as well as emotions and thoughts.[11] When this system functions poorly, it becomes harder to interpret body cues, regulate emotions, and navigate social interactions—challenges that often lie at the heart of emotional and relational distress. Interoceptive disruptions may actively contribute to symptoms rather than just accompany them, helping explain why many diagnoses share features like anxiety, dissociation, and emotional dysregulation,[12] and why individuals with the same diagnosis can present very differently.

Each person's interoceptive patterns are shaped by factors including attachment, stress, trauma, coping styles, and cultural norms. When these processes are disrupted, our sense of connection—to ourselves, to others, and to the world—can be affected. Viewing mental health through this mind–body lens encourages more integrated and compassionate approaches that promote awareness, self-regulation, and healing.

## Synergistic Impacts: When Challenges Combine, the Impacts Multiply

We often think of synergy as something positive—different elements coming together to create greater value. But synergy isn't always beneficial. Consider tragic cases in which people have died from mixing substances; combining drugs can produce effects that are far stronger and more dangerous than taking each one alone.

Challenges that disrupt interoception can be especially serious because they tend to build upon and amplify each other. As discussed earlier, many factors influence interoceptive skills and overall well-being. Here, we examine how attachment disruptions, trauma, stress, and societal norms interact to produce compound—not just additive—effects on interoceptive processing and health.

### *Attachment Disruptions*

Early attachment relationships provide our first experiences of understanding the internal world. In secure relationships, caregivers help children notice, name, and interpret their bodily sensations, which strengthens interoceptive awareness. When attachment is insecure, children receive less consistent support in understanding their internal cues. As a result, their ability to regulate stress and interpret bodily signals may be impaired, creating vulnerabilities that often persist into adulthood.

**Synergistic impacts:** When early attachment disruptions are followed by additional stress or trauma in childhood or adulthood, their effects tend to multiply. This combination doesn't simply add difficulty—it amplifies dysregulation. When early relationships do not provide a stable sense of safety and support, the development of emotion-regulation skills and other internal coping resources can be compromised. Without this foundation, later stress or traumatic experiences are more likely to evoke stronger emotional reactions and less effective ways of coping.

Research suggests that when a person's sense of attachment security has been disrupted, it becomes harder to draw on internal or relational sources of support during times of threat. This reduced capacity for regulation increases vulnerability to ongoing distress and post-traumatic symptoms.[13]

> ***Ava's experience fits this pattern. Growing up with emotionally distant parents and inconsistent caregiving, she never learned to understand or trust her internal cues, leaving her with an unstable foundation for managing emotions and stress. When she was later assaulted by someone she trusted, the emotional impact was intensified. Without a secure internal framework to interpret her feelings, the trauma heightened her emotional reactivity and led her to cope by trying to control her body, engaging in social comparison, and seeking external validation.***

## *Trauma Exposure*

The previous two chapters highlighted the significant strain that trauma places on the interoceptive system and on human functioning in general. Overwhelming or frightening experiences dysregulate the nervous system, making it painful to stay connected to internal cues. States of high activation with a mobilized nervous system, or states of disconnection and shutdown, often become the norm. Sensations may feel confusing, distorted, or even threatening. Many individuals resort to coping strategies like numbing, avoidance, dissociation, or hypervigilance.

Trauma can be especially damaging when it occurs in the context of insecure attachment. When a caregiver either causes trauma or fails to support a child following a traumatic experience, the child lacks someone to help regulate distress.

**Synergistic impacts:** Findings from the original Adverse Childhood Experiences (ACE) Study demonstrate the powerful cumulative effects of adversity. Adults with four or more ACEs face a four- to twelvefold increase in risk for alcohol use disorder, drug addiction, depression, and suicide attempts, and they are more than twice as likely to develop heart disease compared to those with no ACEs.[14]

Childhood trauma also makes it harder to build safe, secure relationships later in life. When caregivers are sources of fear, inconsistency, or harm, the nervous system learns to prioritize self-protection. In adulthood, this can make it difficult to trust others, tolerate emotional vulnerability, or accurately interpret social cues. When these relational challenges combine with interoceptive struggles, the impact is profound. They complicate the ability to regulate emotions, reach out for support, and rely on internal signals to navigate challenges—creating a powerful synergy that heightens overall distress.

*Jason's experience reflects this pattern. Growing up with an abusive, alcoholic father left his nervous system on constant alert. Without a safe adult to help him cope, staying connected to his body now feels confusing and uncomfortable. He swings between being overly activated—angry, reactive, and tense—and shutting down or numbing himself with alcohol. Like many people with high ACE scores, he avoids or suppresses emotions because his internal signals don't feel trustworthy. His trauma history also complicates his relationships, as he often misreads others' intentions. Jason remains stuck in survival mode, struggling to regulate his emotions and trust those around him.*

## *Cultural Norms That Reinforce Disconnection from the Body*

Modern culture makes it easy to disconnect from the inner world. For many, this shows up as a high-stress, productivity-focused mindset that rewards pushing through discomfort and exhaustion while leaving little room for rest or self-regulation. Lifestyle patterns such as poor nutrition, substance use, insufficient sleep, and excessive caffeine intake further strain the system. Digital distractions deepen disconnection from both self and others.

At the same time, how we connect with others has also changed. Working from home, relying on delivery services, and having endless access to entertainment at our fingertips make it easier to limit social interactions. With less community engagement and rising loneliness, people have fewer opportunities for co-regulation and support, making it harder to feel safe with others—and with oneself.

**Synergistic impacts:** When multiple lifestyle challenges arise simultaneously—chronic stress, poor sleep, inadequate nutrition, digital overload, and weakened social ties—their effects tend to compound. In time, these conditions can erode the ability to recognize and interpret bodily signals, pulling us further away from ourselves. Stress may dull awareness, unhealthy habits can disrupt the body's rhythms, and constant distraction can make it harder to notice internal cues. When social support is limited, we also miss key opportunities for co-regulation and recovery. As a result, interoceptive signals may feel muted or confusing, making emotional regulation, clear decision-making, and overall well-being increasingly difficult to sustain.

## Unintended Consequences: When Coping Creates Problems

Sometimes our attempts to solve a problem end up creating new ones. This is especially true when people are coping with trauma, mental health challenges, or ongoing stress. In the face of overwhelming emotions or painful experiences, many individuals lean on strategies that help them get by—disconnecting from others, staying constantly busy, avoiding close relationships, or numbing with substances or behaviors. While these approaches can feel necessary in the moment, they often come with hidden costs. In the long run, the very strategies that once helped someone survive or feel safe can undermine interoceptive awareness, emotional health, and overall well-being.

### *Food as a Coping Tool*

Nearly 45 percent of individuals struggling with weight-related concerns report eating for emotional reasons rather than physiological hunger.[15] While occasional comfort eating is typically harmless, it can become problematic when food becomes a primary means of coping. Research shows that emotional eating is closely linked to disrupted interoception, including difficulty interpreting and trusting bodily signals, as well as fewer emotion regulation skills.[16] When it's hard to distinguish emotional discomfort from physical hunger, food is more often used for relief. Emotional dysregulation and heightened negative feelings also lead to unhealthy eating habits, with stress, body dissatisfaction, low self-esteem, anxiety, and depression all linked to higher levels of emotional eating.[17]

**Unintended consequences:** What often begins as a source of comfort gradually develops into a pattern that complicates the mind–body connection. As concerns about weight grow, they amplify negative feelings such as body dissatisfaction and low self-esteem—emotions that are already difficult to manage. Beyond emotional burdens, obesity also increases health risks like diabetes, heart disease, and musculoskeletal problems, creating a cycle in which emotional and physical challenges continually reinforce each other.

### *Distraction Creates Addiction*

Just as food can serve as a way to cope with overwhelming emotions, other forms of distraction can become powerful yet harmful strategies for managing emotional distress. The MAIA domain that pertains to not distracting oneself reminds us that a tendency to suppress or avoid discomfort can raise stress levels and hinder the use of healthier coping tools. For individuals with trauma histories, attachment wounds, or chronic stress, experiencing intense sensations and emotions can feel nearly impossible. When connecting to bodily sensations feels unsafe or intolerable, distraction through substances or behaviors often becomes a way to escape emotional or physical discomfort—a form of self-medicating distress.

**Unintended consequences:** Using distraction to avoid discomfort can eventually increase vulnerability to addiction. Substances or behaviors may provide quick relief, but they also reinforce the habit of avoiding internal experiences and diminish interoceptive awareness. When the distraction ends, the original distress often returns just as intensely. Addiction then introduces new challenges—declining health, heightened stress, and strained relationships—that can deepen shame and emotional suffering. What initially serves as a coping mechanism can gradually become a cycle where avoidance, distress, and addiction feed into each other.

This is something I often witness in people struggling with substance use disorders, and it is truly heartbreaking. The more life begins to unravel, the more shame and distress they feel, which in turn strengthens the pull toward continued substance use. It becomes a painful cycle that can feel incredibly hard to break.

> *Catherine uses alcohol to escape her relentless self-expectations. Signals such as fatigue or sadness trigger shame, so she stays busy and suppresses her body's cues to keep functioning. While this avoidance reduces distress in the moment, it increases stress and limits healthier coping, leaving her vulnerable to addiction. Wine quickly quiets her inner critic and emotional pain, but the relief is brief. Distress and shame soon return, reinforcing a cycle of avoidance, overwhelm, and drinking that places her at real risk for a substance use disorder.*

### Emotional Avoidance and Disconnection

Emotional avoidance and suppression are common responses among those who have experienced trauma or attachment disruptions. When emotions have been met with danger, judgment, or neglect in the past, shutting them down may seem like the safest and most effective way to cope. Although pushing emotions aside can provide a sense of control or safety, it also comes at a cost—avoiding or suppressing feelings means missing opportunities to connect with the vulnerable parts of oneself that enable meaningful relationships.

**Unintended consequences:** Over time, these protective strategies can unintentionally deepen disconnection from others. Healthy relationships rely on emotional presence—being able to share feelings, seek comfort, and co-regulate with someone trustworthy and reliable. When emotions are suppressed, it becomes harder to communicate needs, ask for support, or let others in. This can leave someone feeling isolated, misunderstood, or alone, even when surrounded by people who care. Emotional avoidance can also increase tension in relationships, reinforcing patterns of stress and withdrawal. Ultimately, the very strategy meant to protect someone from pain can stop them from accessing supportive, co-regulating relationships that foster healing.

> *In Roland's relationships, emotional avoidance and suppression are clearly visible. As a child, he learned that staying emotionally distant was the safest way to cope. As an adult, he maintains a quiet detachment from his family. He avoids conflict, downplays problems, and retreats into work when emotional closeness is needed. While this gives him a sense of control and protects him from vulnerability, it also keeps him disconnected from relationships that could offer comfort and support. With time, his avoidance has increased family tension, damaged relationships, and deepened his feelings of isolation.*

## Pulling the Threads Together—and Preparing for What Comes Next

The challenges people face today—ranging from mental health challenges and chronic illnesses to addiction and unhealthy coping—are deeply interconnected. Disruptions in interoception lie at the core of these struggles, influencing how individuals interpret bodily signals, regulate emotions, handle stress, and relate to themselves and others. When factors like insecure attachment, trauma, cultural expectations, and harmful coping strategies intersect, their effects multiply. What begins as a way to survive or self-soothe can turn into cycles of disconnection, emotional chaos, and suffering as vulnerabilities compound and unintended consequences accumulate.

The remaining chapters in this section build directly on these insights. Each chapter looks at a specific area in which interoceptive disruptions commonly occur, such as anxiety, depression, or physical health challenges. Although each condition has its own distinct features, common themes emerge, including difficulty sensing internal cues or misinterpreting bodily signals.

To support comparisons across conditions, each chapter concludes by highlighting how the MAIA domains may be affected. This structure makes it easier to identify which aspects of interoceptive awareness tend to be impacted by particular conditions or challenges. After outlining these difficulties, the next section introduces tools, strategies, and practices designed to strengthen interoception and support healing.

# 12

# Anxiety Disorders

Throughout my career, one trend has become increasingly clear: Anxiety has risen sharply, especially among young people. This increase isn't caused by a single factor but by a mix of pressures, including constant expectations to perform, the strain of social media, endless comparisons, disrupted sleep, and growing disconnection from others. On a larger scale, people are also living amid increased conflict, economic stress, climate change, racial tensions, and global uncertainty, all while being flooded with information that rarely allows the nervous system to rest.

These conditions shape how we perceive and respond to our inner world. At the same time, this understanding offers hope. By viewing anxiety through the lens of interoception, we can better identify pathways for awareness, support, and resilience, helping people reconnect with their bodies in ways that foster regulation and well-being.

The following are brief definitions of the anxiety disorders covered in this chapter:

- **Generalized anxiety disorder (GAD).** Persistent, excessive worry about everyday life that is difficult to control and often accompanied by physical tension and fatigue.
- **Panic disorder.** Recurrent, unexpected panic attacks characterized by intense fear and physical symptoms, along with ongoing concern about having another attack.
- **Social anxiety disorder.** Intense fear of being judged, embarrassed, or rejected in social or performance settings, leading to avoidance or significant distress.
- **Health anxiety.** Continuous fear or preoccupation with having or developing a serious illness, despite medical reassurance and minimal symptoms.

According to the World Health Organization, anxiety disorders are one of the most common mental health conditions worldwide, with an estimated 4.4 percent of individuals affected as of 2021.[1] Prevalence is highest in high-income countries, including Australia, the United States, and many European nations.[2]

A comprehensive review of anxiety in the United States highlights the prevalence of several common anxiety disorders. The review, published in 2022, indicates that nearly 13 percent of Americans experience an anxiety disorder each year, making anxiety the second most common mental health condition after depression. Social anxiety affects about 13 percent of Americans and is especially common among young people. Just over 6 percent experience GAD, while approximately 5 percent experience panic disorder. Anxiety often occurs alongside physical health issues like heart disease, gastrointestinal disorders, and chronic pain. Despite how widespread anxiety disorders are, most people are not correctly diagnosed, and many with anxiety remain untreated.[3]

## Interoception and Anxiety

Anxiety significantly affects both the body and the mind, and these effects are closely tied to interoceptive processes. When anxiety arises, it activates the body's fight-or-flight response—a survival mechanism designed for real danger but often triggered by perceived threats such as worries or stressful thoughts. When the brain interprets these internal experiences as danger, it prompts the release of stress hormones, including adrenaline and cortisol, leading to physical changes such as a racing heart, muscle tension, and increased alertness. With time, repeated activation of this response can leave the body stuck in a state of chronic arousal.

Anxiety also shapes how we think. It often leads to rumination—repetitive, looping thoughts about potential threats, past mistakes, or what-if scenarios. This constant mental replay can exaggerate perceived danger and undermine confidence in one's ability to cope, creating a cycle in which bodily sensations and anxious thoughts feed into one another.

Because anxiety engages the stress response, it produces a wide range of interoceptive cues across bodily systems, including

- **Cardiovascular:** rapid heartbeat, palpitations, chest tightness, elevated blood pressure
- **Respiratory:** short or rapid breathing, difficulty breathing, choking sensation, lump in the throat

- **Gastrointestinal:** stomach aches, "butterflies," nausea, vomiting, diarrhea, constipation, indigestion, loss of appetite
- **Musculoskeletal:** muscle tension, stiffness, soreness, teeth grinding, jaw clenching
- **Sensory:** dizziness, light-headedness, headaches, shakiness, tingling or numbness, feeling faint
- **Autonomic:** restlessness, jitteriness, internal vibrations, heightened startle reflex, feeling detached from the body

## Interoceptive Disruptions in Anxiety

There are several significant ways that anxiety can disrupt or hijack interoceptive processes. In this section, you will notice many of the themes that appeared in earlier chapters. You may also recognize some of these descriptions in your own experiences—and wonder whether there's something different you could do. The good news is that there is: The last section introduces tools for enhancing interoceptive awareness and the mind–body connection. But first, here are some of the altered patterns that are specific to anxiety.

### *Hyperattention to Sensations*

Research shows that people with generalized anxiety disorder, panic disorder, and social anxiety disorder are all more aware of their internal bodily signals—such as heartbeat, breathing, or physical tension—than those without anxiety. This heightened awareness manifests differently depending on the disorder. In GAD, individuals tend to monitor their bodily sensations broadly and continually, reflecting their ongoing and generalized worry. Those with panic disorder, on the other hand, become sharply focused on specific physiological changes linked to fear, for example, a racing heart or shortness of breath.[4] By contrast, people with social anxiety disorder often focus their attention inward during social situations. They become more aware of sensations like a racing heart, blushing, or sweating, and believe these reactions affect how others see them.[5]

Health anxiety occurs when everyday bodily sensations feel threatening, even without medical cause. This largely automatic response puts the brain into a "better safe than sorry" mode, where stress and constant monitoring lead to *somatic amplification*—normal sensations are experienced as stronger and more alarming. As attention increases, sensations intensify, reinforcing a cycle of worry, body scanning, and rising anxiety.[6]

*Hailey's early experiences of physical vulnerability and her mother's anxious monitoring taught her to stay alert for potential danger. This mindset drives her to constantly check her body and seek reassurance, which in turn amplifies her sensations and anxiety. The ongoing cycle keeps her stress response activated, making her symptoms feel worse. While she is highly aware of her body, this awareness is marked by fear and mistrust.*

Overall, although these disorders all involve increased focus on internal sensations, they differ in how that awareness is experienced and interpreted. These patterns reflect the unique nature of each anxiety condition. Often, heightened body awareness is not paired with emotional understanding, making sensations feel confusing or alarming, which increases distress rather than providing clarity or insight.

## *Misinterpretation of Bodily Signals*

Ideally, noticing bodily sensations involves a calm, flexible awareness of the body without excessive focus or alarm. Sensations like heartbeats, fatigue, muscle tension, warmth, or brief discomfort naturally come and go, often registering in the background while attention stays mostly on daily activities. But across anxiety disorders, a different pattern emerges: Individuals tend to overmonitor their internal cues and misinterpret their bodily sensations, which fuels and sustains anxious states. This misinterpretation often occurs as people try to explain a bodily change (e.g., "Why is my heart racing?") or assign it meaning (e.g., "Does this mean I'm in danger?"). When these processes become altered, benign physiological signals are reinterpreted as threats, amplifying emotional distress and leading to maladaptive coping.

In panic disorder, internal sensations are often misinterpreted in negative or catastrophic ways—ordinary bodily sensations are viewed as dangerous.[7] For instance, a rapid heartbeat or shortness of breath may be mistaken for signs of a heart attack. These catastrophic beliefs heighten vigilance and intensify worry, creating a self-reinforcing cycle of anxiety and panic.

In GAD, misreading bodily cues tends to be subtler but more continuous and ongoing. People can stay highly tuned in to their internal sensations, often experiencing them as more important or intense than they actually are. When the cause of these sensations is unclear (e.g., "Why does my stomach feel tight?"), the ambiguity can lead to repeated, worry-driven interpretations. As a result, even ordinary changes in the body can become linked to persistent anxious thoughts.[8]

For people with social anxiety disorder, bodily sensations are often misinterpreted in ways that fuel fears of being judged. During social situations, individuals may become very aware of a racing heart, blushing, or sweating and believe that others can see these signs, viewing them as "evidence" that they are incompetent, awkward, or flawed.[9] These interpretations heighten anxiety and make interactions seem more threatening than they actually are.

In health anxiety, bodily sensations are often misinterpreted, with attention narrowing around fears of illness. People may become selectively focused on physical cues that seem to signal a health problem, sometimes noticing symptoms even when none are objectively present. This heightened vigilance and tendency to catastrophize bodily sensations reinforce anxiety and help sustain the cycle of health-related worry.[10]

## *Distraction and Avoidance*

As we've discussed, we live in a culture of constant distraction. From endless scrolling to overeating or substance use, there are countless ways to numb or avoid what we feel. While these behaviors may offer brief comfort, they often do more harm than good. Avoiding difficult emotions or bodily sensations might bring short-term relief, but it also prevents the development of healthier coping strategies.

When anxiety becomes overwhelming, it makes sense that some individuals seek a break from it by seeking out something that numbs. This can show up as emotional avoidance or strong urges to distract through scrolling, eating, or substance use. Although distraction may temporarily dampen anxiety, it also blocks opportunities to regulate the nervous system in more adaptive ways. This can trap people in a repetitive cycle—swinging from intense anxiety to avoidance or shutdown, then back to anxiety once the distraction ends. Over time, this pattern makes it harder to access nervous system regulation, connection, and effective self-care. In short, distraction may feel protective, but it can ultimately keep people stuck and disconnected from the resources that support healing.

This avoidance pattern is reflected in the close link between anxiety and substance use disorders (SUDs). A 2015 analysis of global studies reports that individuals with an alcohol use disorder were 2.1 times more likely to have an anxiety disorder than nonusers.[11] A large US-based survey of more than forty-three thousand adults found that almost 18 percent of individuals with a substance use disorder also had an anxiety disorder. The connection is even stronger with specific diagnoses: Nearly half of those with PTSD also meet criteria for a SUD, and GAD is also strongly associated with substance use, as many people attempt to self-medicate their anxiety with drugs or alcohol.[12]

Although substances may seem to provide quick relief, they often create a painful cycle. Alcohol or cannabis can briefly numb the uncomfortable bodily sensations of anxiety, but as the effects wear off, the anxiety and discomfort return—often more intensely—leading to repeated use. Eventually, anxiety and substance use begin to reinforce each other, with each making the other harder to control. We will explore this relationship more thoroughly in a later chapter.

*Catherine is high-functioning and may not seem anxious, but worry is constant in her daily life. She appears calm and capable, yet underneath, ongoing anxiety persists. She overprepares—rechecking work, rehearsing conversations, planning ahead—viewing it as responsibility. When tension builds, she uses alcohol to calm her mind. Her anxiety doesn't limit her ability to function; it fuels it. Perfectionism and fear of judgment keep her nervous system in constant overdrive, hiding anxiety behind competence. While alcohol provides brief relief, it disrupts healthier regulation and raises the likelihood that her anxiety will worsen with time.*

Avoidance can also show up in subtle, everyday ways. One increasingly common form involves the overuse of digital technology—something many of us engage in at times. Scrolling through social media, watching videos, or chatting online can offer quick relief by distracting us from distressing thoughts, emotions, or bodily sensations. Technology may also be used to postpone tasks or situations that provoke anxiety. Research suggests that this kind of digital engagement can function as a form of experiential avoidance. For example, one study found that problematic smartphone use is linked to higher levels of avoidance and anxiety.[13] This indicates that technology can sometimes serve as a way to step back from uncomfortable internal experiences.

Although digital distraction might feel comforting in the moment, it often reinforces avoidance. Instead of learning to tolerate or work through anxiety, people learn to escape it. In time, this reliance on technology can make it harder to face challenges directly and may even increase anxiety.

Food can serve a similar function. Individuals with GAD, for example, frequently engage in emotional eating—consuming food not out of physical hunger but to manage feelings of worry, tension, or distress. Eating, particularly sugary or high-fat foods, can temporarily ease anxiety by triggering pleasurable brain responses. However, this learned association between negative emotions and eating can become automatic and difficult to break. In the long term, emotional eating is linked to undesirable weight gain, guilt, shame, and even eating disorders. It traps individuals in a cycle where negative emotions lead to eating, which then produces more negative feelings about one's body or self-control.[14]

### *Rumination*

Rumination is the tendency to dwell on repetitive, negative thoughts. It is common in generalized anxiety disorder (as well as depression, OCD, and PTSD, which we'll explore in other chapters). Research shows that rumination doesn't just affect mental health on its own but also interacts in important ways with interoceptive awareness. One study found that people who ruminated often *and* had poor interoceptive awareness reported the highest levels of anxiety and depression. This suggests that when someone is less attuned to their internal bodily cues, their negative thought patterns may exert an even stronger influence on their emotions, exacerbating distress.[15] While rumination alone is associated with emotional suffering, the combination of repetitive negative thinking and low body awareness appears especially detrimental.

At the same time, ruminators who focus intensely on their internal states—who may be overly aware of their bodies—can face a different challenge: Increased interoception can heighten emotional experiences, making negative feelings feel more intense and overwhelming. This emotional intensification can, in turn, disrupt clear thinking and problem-solving, especially under stress, creating a vicious cycle in which negative thoughts and heightened emotions reinforce each other. This pattern gradually makes it more difficult to regulate mood or respond effectively to challenges.[16]

## Predictive Processing

As a reminder, predictive processing is the brain's energy-efficient way of understanding the world by anticipating what will happen rather than simply reacting. It uses past experiences to estimate how our body and senses *should* feel, then compares those guesses to reality and adjusts if necessary. When predictions don't match reality—known as *prediction errors*—ideally, the brain updates them with new learning that more closely reflects what is happening.

With anxiety, prediction errors often don't get updated, or the predictions themselves are inaccurate because of overestimating danger or misreading body signals. Sometimes this occurs when the brain misinterprets normal sensations as signs of threat. For example, when someone with social anxiety notices they're sweating during a conversation, they may assume others will notice and judge them, which increases anxiety and sweating. In reality, the other person usually doesn't notice at all. Because the brain's guess doesn't match the actual cause, the mismatch fuels more anxiety, reinforcing the false belief that something is wrong.

One way this plays out is through avoidance, which keeps anxiety stuck instead of allowing predictions to be updated. Someone with social anxiety might predict, "If I go to that party, I'll embarrass myself and everyone will judge me." If they avoid going, their brain never gathers evidence to challenge that belief—perhaps people would have been welcoming, or the conversation might have gone smoothly. Without new information, the prediction remains unchanged, and the anxiety stays just as strong. Eventually, this cycle of avoidance reinforces the original belief and makes future social situations feel just as threatening, preventing the brain from learning that its prediction may be inaccurate.

## How MAIA Domains Can Be Impacted in Anxiety Disorders

Anxiety disorders often involve heightened attention to specific bodily signals—such as breathing, heart rate, or blushing—paired with overly negative evaluations of these sensations and difficulty using interoception for regulation. These patterns vary across individuals and anxiety disorder types, but several MAIA domains tend to be affected. Here are some of the common ways interoception may be altered, based on the MAIA framework.

**Noticing.** The noticing of distressing bodily signals is often heightened in individuals with anxiety disorders, but this attention is typically narrow and unbalanced. While the MAIA "noticing" domain reflects a broad, inclusive awareness of bodily sensations—neutral, positive, and uncomfortable—anxiety tends to draw attention mainly toward sensations associated with the stress response, such as a rapid heartbeat or gastrointestinal discomfort. As a result, increased noticing can amplify distress rather than promote understanding. Some individuals experience the opposite pattern: Anxious thoughts pull attention away from bodily sensations altogether, or they may notice their bodies only when sensations become intense.

**Not-Worrying.** This domain reflects the ability to remain calm in response to bodily sensations such as pain or discomfort. People with anxiety are often more sensitive to internal cues they find unpleasant or worrying, and they may catastrophize these sensations. Neutral or ambiguous body signals can also be perceived as signs that something is wrong. This combination—heightened body awareness and a tendency to interpret bodily sensations negatively—plays a central role in the development and maintenance of anxiety disorders.

**Self-Regulation.** This domain centers on the capacity to use bodily sensations to guide emotional and behavioral responses in healthy ways, such as grounding or calming oneself. For individuals with anxiety, bodily cues may feel less like supportive resources and more like overwhelming signals of distress, such as a racing heart or tightness in the chest. This heightened focus on anxious sensations can make it harder to self-soothe, contributing to greater emotional dysregulation and, over time, intensifying anxiety symptoms.

# 13
# Depression

Depression is among the most common mental health conditions worldwide and remains the leading cause of disability globally.[1] In 2024, about 8.2 percent of Americans aged eighteen or older experienced a major depressive episode in the previous year.[2] Across Europe, the rates of depression among adults vary widely from 2.56 percent in Slovakia to much higher levels in more affluent nations such as Germany (9.24 percent) and Portugal (9.15 percent).[3]

Depression doesn't present only as sadness or low mood. It also involves changes in sleep, appetite, energy, motivation, and physical health. Increasingly, researchers and clinicians recognize that depression is not solely a problem of the mind or mood—it emerges when communication between the body and the brain is altered.[4]

People living with major depressive disorder (MDD) often experience a deep sense of emptiness, hopelessness, or a loss of interest in activities that once brought them joy. But depression isn't only emotional; it frequently shows up physically as well. Many individuals notice changes in appetite or weight, disrupted sleep, persistent fatigue or low energy, and significant shifts in movement, such as restlessness or slowed behavior. These physical symptoms commonly appear alongside feelings of worthlessness, difficulty concentrating, or recurring thoughts about death or suicide.

In depression, interoceptive processes are altered in various ways: sometimes muted, sometimes overwhelming, and often unreliable. These disruptions can cause confusion, disconnection, or sensory overload. This chapter explores how disrupted mind–body communication underlies many of depression's core symptoms.

Depression, like the other mental health conditions discussed in this book, is not simply "in the head." It reflects a breakdown in body–brain communication—one that can leave individuals estranged from their internal experience, flooded by it, or unable to use it to regulate their emotions. Viewing depression through the lens of interoception offers a new way to understand its symptoms and the far-reaching impact it has on those who live with it.

## The Body's Role in Depression

Depression affects nearly every bodily system that communicates with the brain. While anxiety often activates the body into a state of hyperarousal, depression tends to slow it down, changing how internal signals are generated, perceived, and interpreted. This altered interoceptive landscape means that many physical sensations linked to depression—from fatigue and pain to digestive discomfort—become central to how individuals experience the condition. Here's how depression influences some of the bodily systems discussed earlier in this book.

### CARDIOVASCULAR SYSTEM

- Elevated blood pressure and heart rate, increasing cardiovascular disease risk.[5]
- Heightened awareness of heartbeat sensations (e.g., racing, skipped beats, chest tightness), which is frequently mistaken for anxiety or panic.

### IMMUNE SYSTEM

- Increased immune activity and inflammation.[6]
- Inflammation triggers interoceptive signals like aches, malaise, and diffuse pain.

### NERVOUS SYSTEM

- Structural and functional changes in the brain—particularly in the hippocampus and amygdala—impair emotional regulation and cognition.[7]
- Symptoms include brain fog, poor memory, and reduced concentration.
- Widespread neurotransmitter dysregulation, especially involving serotonin, dopamine, and norepinephrine, disrupts mood, motivation, cognition, and stress response.[8]

GASTROINTESTINAL SYSTEM

- Disrupted digestive processes are common, leading to nausea, bloating, abdominal discomfort, constipation, and irritable bowel symptoms.[9]
- Significant shifts in appetite can occur, resulting in weight loss or gain.

THE GUT–BRAIN CONNECTION

- Depression is frequently associated with imbalances in the gut microbial community, known as *dysbiosis*.[10]
- The gut microbiome regulates key neurotransmitters, including serotonin (over 80 percent of which is produced in the gut) and GABA.[11] Disruptions can impair emotional regulation and alter interoceptive feedback, reinforcing depressive states.
- Digestive signals and emotional states interact in a feedback loop, each influencing the other.

## Fatigue

A study by Michael Eggart and colleagues examined how fatigue, motivation, and behavior are closely linked in depression, highlighting the body's central role in this relationship. Fatigue is one of the most common and disruptive symptoms of depression. People often experience profound low energy, heaviness, poor concentration, and a lack of motivation. Unlike ordinary tiredness, this fatigue doesn't improve with rest. Eggart's team suggests that these symptoms stem from disruptions in interoception.[12]

Typically, the brain uses predictive processing to maintain bodily balance, anticipating what the body needs and updating those predictions in response to internal signals. In depression, this system breaks down: The brain's predictions and the body's actual state no longer align, creating persistent prediction errors that reflect failed attempts to restore equilibrium. This mismatch leaves individuals feeling exhausted even after they've had enough rest.

Over time, persistent fatigue can erode motivation and deepen feelings of helplessness and discouragement, leading people to believe that their actions cannot influence their emotional state. This bodily mistrust can extend beyond physical sensations, reinforcing hopelessness and fueling withdrawal. The study also found that paying attention to bodily sensations can be a double-edged sword. While some awareness may support energy and focus, paying too much attention to discomfort can worsen fatigue by amplifying negative sensations and consuming mental resources. These patterns form a self-perpetuating cycle in which fatigue, low motivation, and behavior continually shape one another. They illustrate how depression alters bodily experience, emphasizing that it is as much a physical condition as it is a psychological one.[13]

## Anxious Depression—The Other Side of the Coin

The previous section emphasizes major depressive disorder as an experience marked by fatigue and disconnection that feels heavy and overwhelming. But this does not reflect the experience of everyone who struggles with depression. For many, the lived experience looks very different.

The DSM-5 includes an *anxious distress specifier* that describes a form of MDD involving significant anxiety. Symptoms include feeling tense or "on edge," being unusually restless, having trouble focusing due to worry, fearing that something terrible might happen, or feeling a sense of losing control. Anxious distress often involves physical agitation that reflects heightened nervous system activation. Common signs include restlessness, fidgeting, a racing heart, and gastrointestinal discomfort. People with anxious distress tend to face greater challenges, such as more significant daily impairment and reduced responsiveness to standard treatments, compared to those who have depression without substantial anxiety.[14] Researchers have also found that this form of "anxious depression" is common, impacting an estimated 45 to 55 percent of people with depression.[15]

Anxious depression's most defining feature is the range and severity of physical symptoms that accompany the depressive state. Unlike typical MDD, which tends to present more with emotional and cognitive symptoms, anxious depression involves increased bodily arousal and more physical signs of anxiety. These include heart palpitations, excessive sweating, trembling, and respiratory issues such as shortness of breath, chest tightness, or a feeling of not getting enough air. Gastrointestinal problems are also prevalent, ranging from nausea and abdominal discomfort to bloating, appetite changes, and disrupted digestion. Many individuals also report muscle tension, headaches, restlessness, and a general sense of bodily unease—clear signs of how anxiety affects the physical experience.

Physical discomfort is often accompanied by health-related anxiety and panic-like episodes, which further distinguish anxious depression from non-anxious forms.[16] People may fixate on bodily sensations, misinterpreting them as signs of serious illness, or experience sudden surges of fear, a racing heart, and a sense of losing control—experiences similar to panic attacks. These intense bodily symptoms can result in more frequent doctor visits and increased avoidance behaviors aimed at reducing anxiety.

***Although Hailey exhibits a pattern of worry and misinterprets harmless physical sensations, she does not show consistent depressive symptoms. However, she is at an increased risk of transitioning from primarily anxiety-based symptoms to fuller depressive symptoms.***

While physiological activation dominates the clinical picture, anxious depression also involves greater cognitive disruption and emotional reactivity than typical MDD. Concentration difficulties, mental fog, and decision-making challenges are common and can significantly impair daily life.[17] These difficulties likely stem from increased rumination and hypervigilance, as anxious thoughts consume mental resources and make it harder to focus on cognitive tasks. Emotional responses also tend to be more reactive, characterized by increased irritability, agitation, and sensitivity to stress. Together, these features create a multidimensional condition in which anxiety's influence on the body amplifies mental and emotional disturbances, forming a distinctive and particularly challenging depressive syndrome.

## The Nervous System and Depression

Looking at depression through the lens of the nervous system helps explain why it manifests so differently across individuals. In depression without anxiety, the body often shifts into a low-energy, slowed-down state marked by fatigue, withdrawal, emotional numbness, and reduced awareness of the bodily signals that normally foster motivation and engagement. This pattern reflects the nervous system's attempt to cope when stress feels overwhelming or unchangeable, but it can also leave people feeling disconnected from themselves and the world around them.

In anxious depression, the picture is more complex. Rather than settling into a single state, the nervous system may oscillate between increased activation and shutdown. This can produce a distressing mix of agitation, worry, physical tension, and exhaustion—where the body feels both *too activated* and *shut down* simultaneously. From this standpoint, the differences between depression and anxious depression are not contradictions; they represent distinct bodily responses to ongoing stress rather than opposing conditions.

## Comorbidity: When Interoceptive Miscommunication Spreads

Comorbidity refers to having more than one disorder or condition at the same time. Depression rarely occurs alone. For many people, it co-occurs with other mental health conditions—such as anxiety disorders, substance use disorders, or PTSD—as well as a range of chronic physical illnesses. These overlapping conditions often make depression more severe, harder to treat, and more disruptive to daily life, while also increasing the risk of suicidal behavior.

Among mental health conditions, anxiety disorders are the most common co-occurring diagnoses, affecting up to 58 percent of individuals with depression.[18] Research also shows that in as many as 68 percent of those with both anxiety and depression, anxiety symptoms appear first.[19] Substance use disorders, particularly alcohol dependence, are also frequently present alongside depression, impacting nearly half of women and a quarter of men with alcohol-related issues. Substance use can mask depressive symptoms. These comorbid conditions further increase suffering—they worsen symptoms, slow recovery, and reduce the chances of following through with treatment.[20]

People with depression are also more likely to develop heart disease, stroke, diabetes, chronic pain, obesity, and cancer.[21] Interoception helps explain why these conditions so often cluster together. When communication between the body and brain is disrupted, signals related to stress, pain, fatigue, and emotion become harder to interpret and regulate. In time, this strain can extend beyond mental health.

Comorbid disorders are not coincidental. They reflect how disruptions in bodily awareness and regulation can spread across emotional, behavioral, and physical systems, reinforcing the idea that depression is not just a mood disorder but a broader breakdown in body–brain communication.

## General Interoceptive Disruptions in Depression

Next is a summary of some of the interoceptive disruptions commonly seen in depression and anxious depression. You may notice that the list overlaps with the general interoceptive disruptions discussed in the previous chapter on anxiety disorders.

### *Hyperattention to and Misinterpretation of Body Sensations*

People with depression or anxious depression often experience disturbances in how they attend to and interpret bodily signals. They may become overly focused on internal sensations such as heartbeat, breathing, pain, or fatigue. In depression, this hyperattention is often directed toward somatic symptoms like pain or exhaustion, which can heighten emotional distress and reinforce negative mood states. One study even found that paying excessive attention to the body can exacerbate fatigue.[22]

In anxious depression, this heightened focus is typically more pronounced and mirrors patterns seen in anxiety disorders. Individuals become highly sensitive to bodily cues and may misinterpret normal sensations, such as a rapid heartbeat or shortness of breath, as signs of danger or illness.

Even when the body provides accurate signals, the brain may interpret them negatively. In depression, ordinary sensations may be viewed as signs of weakness or failure. In anxious depression, the same sensations are more likely to be interpreted as indicators of danger. Eventually, these interpretations increase anxiety, contribute to depressed mood, and create a cycle in which everyday body sensations become a constant source of distress. Importantly, this isn't a matter of choice. The mind can automatically lock onto the body in both depression and anxious depression, and that attention naturally amplifies what's felt.

At the core of both conditions is a combination of unclear or unreliable bodily signals and an overly strong, distressing reaction to those sensations.[23] Not only are bodily cues often misread or intensified, but the emotional response to them is heightened, further fueling the painful cycle of hyperattention, misinterpretation, and emotional suffering.

### *Avoidance and Distraction in Response to Bodily Sensations*

People with depression or anxious depression often try to manage uncomfortable physical or emotional feelings by avoiding them or distracting themselves—a pattern similar to what we see in anxiety disorders. While these strategies can provide short-term relief, over time they weaken the ability to tune into internal experience, making it harder to notice and interpret body signals and emotions. In depression, this may appear as emotional numbness, withdrawal, or a sense of disconnection from the body.

In anxious depression, avoidance often pairs with hypervigilance. People may become acutely aware of uncomfortable physical sensations when stressed, then try to escape or shut them down once they feel overwhelming. Many turn to distractions like social media, food, or substances to cope. Although these habits may feel soothing at first, people can come to rely on them for emotional relief.

Research by Zahir Vally and colleagues, for example, found that individuals with depression are more likely to develop problematic social media use, turning to online platforms for comfort or connection when feeling sad or out of control.[24] Similarly, high rates of co-occurring substance use disorders among individuals with depression and anxious depression suggest attempts to dull or escape overwhelming interoceptive and emotional experiences.[25]

Although these coping strategies may ease discomfort in the moment, they often reinforce fear of bodily sensations and prevent people from learning that these sensations are tolerable and safe. In the long term, this cycle sustains depression, increases fear of future discomfort, and further disconnects the body from emotion—ironically making the very distress that people seek to avoid harder to manage.

### *Rumination and Worry*

In depression, rumination and worry center on a deeply negative view of oneself. People often see themselves as flawed or defective and focus on evidence that seems to confirm this belief, such as critical feedback or painful memories. They may feel like a burden in relationships, withdraw socially, and lose a sense of belonging—patterns that further reinforce a negative self-image. A key feature is self-focused attention. People spend significant time thinking about themselves and struggle to stay present. Even when they try, their thoughts tend to revert to repetitive rumination about the past or worry about the future.[26]

These persistent thought patterns can disrupt awareness of current bodily sensations, replacing it with a top-down cognitive focus fueled by cognitive distortions. In some cases, as in anxious depression, rumination mixes with worry and bodily scanning, causing people to become hyperfocused on internal signals, interpret them negatively, and struggle to regulate their responses.

*David's experience illustrates this pattern. A harsh self-view and constant rumination drive his depression. He blames his struggles on personal flaws and fixates on past mistakes or negative feedback, reinforcing the belief that he's a failure. Feeling like a burden, he withdraws from relationships, deepening his isolation and hopelessness. Even when he's with others, his attention quickly turns inward, trapping him in a cycle of negative, repetitive thinking that keeps him stuck.*

### *Blunted Interoceptive Awareness Leading to Blunted Motivation*

Many people with depression feel disconnected from their bodies and struggle to sense or interpret internal signals. Without clear access to these signals, they may feel emotionally numb and find it hard to recognize what they are feeling and why. This tendency is closely linked to interoception: When internal signals are muted, distorted, or difficult to interpret, emotional responses can become blunted or harder to regulate, contributing to feelings of emptiness, disconnection, or overwhelming sadness.

This diminished bodily awareness also interferes with everyday functioning. Internal signals typically motivate behavior and guide decision-making, but when they are dulled, maintaining routines or taking action becomes more challenging. For example, missing cues such as hunger or low energy can disrupt daily structure, while difficulty sensing emotional needs can reduce motivation to seek support or engage in therapy. As a result, people may struggle to recognize what they need or when to act, weakening follow-through and making it harder to build healthy habits or stay engaged in treatment.[27]

Interoceptive signals also influence how we assess risk and respond to stress. When these signals are muted, individuals may misjudge danger or fail to respond protectively. Someone with depression, for instance, may delay seeking medical care because the emotional urgency that would normally prompt action is diminished. As depression deepens, this disconnection from the body can become more pronounced.

Julie Dunne and colleagues describe how, over the course of a major depressive episode, individuals may gradually stop listening to bodily sensations until they stop noticing them altogether, losing access to the body-based cues that support emotional awareness and self-regulation.[28] With time, this erosion of interoceptive awareness can further impair motivation, emotional clarity, and decision-making, reducing the body's ability to support healthy behavior and emotional well-being.

## How MAIA Domains Can Be Impacted in Depression

Depression doesn't just affect mood or motivation; it profoundly alters communication between mind and body, as seen in several domains of the MAIA framework.

**Trust.** This is a key aspect of interoceptive awareness that is significantly affected in moderate to severe depression. Low scores suggest that depressed individuals feel less confident in trusting their bodies, which can reduce confidence in interpreting internal signals. Simply put, the more depressed someone feels, the less likely they are to trust cues like hunger, fatigue, or physical tension. Dunne and colleagues propose that this loss of bodily trust may be one of the earliest ways depression impacts the connection with the body, making internal sensations harder to interpret or rely on.[29] For those with anxious depression, bodily messages are harder to trust because they signal stronger warnings; the body often feels unsafe due to overexperiencing and overinterpreting danger cues.

**Noticing.** This domain reflects overall awareness of bodily sensations and is often diminished in moderate to severe depression. Many people perceive body signals as quieter or more difficult to detect, which can lead to a sense of disconnection from their inner experience. When bodily awareness decreases, emotions may also seem muted or unclear, since physical sensations help shape emotional understanding. This pattern overlaps with alexithymia in depression, where difficulty identifying emotions is partly linked to reduced awareness of the body's cues. Conversely, those with anxious depression may notice sensations but tend to focus on signals that indicate discomfort or threat, while neutral or comfortable sensations are overlooked.

**Emotional Awareness.** This domain reflects how well a person can connect bodily sensations with emotional experiences. People with moderate to severe depression often struggle to make this connection, contributing to emotional detachment and alexithymia, which is common in depression. Research suggests this breakdown may develop over time: As trust in bodily sensations decreases, individuals may become less likely to notice or listen to their bodies.[30] This can eventually increase the sense of disconnection from the body's signals that typically support emotional awareness and intensify the numbness and detachment often associated with depression.

# 14

# OCD and Related Disorders

Conditions such as obsessive-compulsive disorder (OCD), nonsuicidal self-injury (NSSI), body dysmorphic disorder (BDD), muscle dysmorphia (MD), and skin-picking disorder (also known as excoriation disorder) can be understood as part of a broader OCD-related spectrum.[1] What connects them is a shared difficulty with interoceptive and self-regulation processes. Together, they reflect a common underlying pattern: struggles with interpreting, regulating, or soothing internal sensations and emotional discomfort. To cope with tension or distress, individuals with these challenges often engage in repetitive behaviors, such as checking, picking, exercising, or self-injury, to reduce discomfort or regain a sense of control.

The DSM-5 groups OCD with related conditions like body dysmorphic disorder (including muscle dysmorphia; both are discussed later in this chapter) and skin-picking disorder because they share similar repetitive, ritual-like patterns of behavior and mental focus. Some researchers have also shown that NSSI aligns with this pattern.[2] Although it may look different on the surface, it serves a similar function: managing overwhelming inner sensations or emotions. If you've ever felt compelled to repeatedly do something to quiet an unbearable feeling or sensation, this framework may help you make sense of that experience.

In this chapter, we explore how these conditions reflect a shared mind–body cycle. Internal sensations are experienced as uncomfortable or urgent, which naturally triggers distress and leads to repeated behaviors that provide brief relief. In time, these responses can make it harder to trust or accurately interpret bodily signals, leaving individuals stuck in patterns of ineffective self-regulation. OCD-related behaviors aren't only about intrusive thoughts or habits; they also reflect how the body's signals are perceived, understood, and responded to.

## Obsessive-Compulsive Disorder

The DSM-5 defines obsessive-compulsive disorder (OCD) as a condition in which individuals experience unwanted, distressing thoughts, urges, or images (called *obsessions*). They also feel compelled to perform repetitive behaviors or mental rituals (called *compulsions*) to reduce anxiety or prevent harm they believe might occur if they do not carry out these actions.[3] These behaviors often consume a considerable amount of time and interfere with daily functioning. Even though many people with OCD recognize that their fears or actions are unreasonable, and may even increase distress, the urges are often too strong to resist, reinforcing a cycle of anxiety followed by short-term relief.

In OCD, distress isn't limited to intrusive thoughts; it is also closely connected to what is happening in the body. Many of the urges and sensations that drive compulsive behaviors arise from disruptions in interoceptive processing and are experienced in three main ways: sensory phenomena, premonitory urges, and disgust proneness.

### *Sensory Phenomena*

Many people with OCD experience symptoms that are not driven primarily by fear or anxiety but by uncomfortable internal sensations known as *sensory phenomena*. These sensations, reported by about 65 percent of people with OCD,[4] can manifest as a persistent "not-just-right" feeling, a sense of incompleteness, or visceral urges such as feeling "dirty" that prompt repetitive washing, checking, or organizing behaviors. These actions are attempts to fix an internal sense of "wrongness." For instance, clothing or bodily sensations may feel "not right" unless items are repeatedly adjusted—socks aligned perfectly or tags lying flat. Similarly, misaligned objects can create an internal sense of discomfort that drives a person to arrange them until symmetry feels correct. These behaviors aren't aimed at stopping something bad from happening; rather, they're about calming bodily discomfort when things don't feel right.

Skin-picking disorder is an OCD-related behavior in which a person repeatedly picks at their skin, often resulting in skin damage and significant emotional distress. The behavior is frequently triggered by uncomfortable bodily sensations, such as tension, itching, or a feeling that something is not quite right.[5] Picking is usually followed by a temporary sense of relief. Many episodes occur automatically or out of habit and are influenced more by bodily cues than by conscious emotional intent. For example, someone might absentmindedly touch their face, notice a small bump, and feel a strong urge to remove it. Picking may continue until the area feels more settled, showing that the behavior is driven by sensory cues and a need for the body to feel "complete," rather than an intention to harm oneself.

Researchers link these experiences to disrupted interoception. People with OCD who encounter sensory phenomena tend to be more easily distracted or distressed by internal bodily sensations.[6] Altered interoceptive processing may cause otherwise ordinary sensations to feel amplified, misinterpreted, or intolerable. In these cases, distress is not driven by fears of harm or contamination but by a persistent sense that something feels off or out of balance in the body. Repetitive behaviors function as attempts to restore a subjective sense of comfort or "rightness."

## *Premonitory Urges*

Premonitory urges are uncomfortable internal sensations that build up before a movement or compulsion. They are often felt as rising tension, pressure, or itchy or tingling sensations that ease only after the action is performed. These urges are common in tic disorders and help explain why certain behaviors can feel so hard to resist.[7]

In tic disorders, urges typically arise in a specific body part and tend to subside once the tic occurs. In OCD, similar sensations are more often diffuse and show up as a general feeling that something is unfinished or "not quite right," rather than being tied to a particular spot in the body.[8] In both cases, these urges reflect differences in how the body senses and interprets internal signals. When those signals feel uncomfortable or out of balance, the urge to act becomes stronger as the body seeks relief.

In OCD, internal discomfort often builds until a compulsion is performed, followed by brief relief. While this pattern resembles what happens in tic disorders, a key distinction is that tics are involuntary, whereas compulsions are intentional actions aimed at reducing discomfort or restoring a sense of order.[9] For example, someone may know they locked the door but still feel rising tension in their body until they check again and feel temporary ease.

These urges may represent exaggerated versions of everyday bodily signals that guide normal actions like blinking or scratching an itch.[10] In OCD, however, these signals become amplified and harder to regulate, making action feel like the only way to ease the discomfort—even though the relief is short-lived.

### *Disgust Proneness*

Contamination OCD involves persistent worries about germs, dirt, or spreading contamination to oneself or others. To manage these fears, people often feel compelled to wash, clean, or sanitize repeatedly. This form of OCD is closely tied to disgust—a natural emotion meant to protect us from illness. In contamination OCD, that disgust response becomes overly sensitive, producing strong bodily sensations such as nausea, revulsion, or an internal feeling of being "dirty," even when no real danger is present.

Interoceptive functioning plays a key role in disgust proneness—how strongly someone reacts to sensations they find disgusting. This includes both how easily disgust is triggered (disgust propensity) and how distressing or uncomfortable the feeling becomes once it arises (disgust sensitivity).[11] For example, someone might feel nauseated or gag just by thinking about bodily fluids. If that reaction becomes overwhelming, it can quickly trigger urges to avoid, wash, or eliminate the sensation.

Strong disgust responses are closely linked to contamination-related OCD. A person might dispose of items they believe are contaminated, even when the actual risk is low. Contamination can be physical—such as contact with germs or dirt—or mental, like feeling internally dirty or tainted without any external contact. While washing may help with physical contamination, it often doesn't relieve mental contamination, which stems from internal sensations of disgust rather than actual dirt or germs.

Research shows that disgust is a basic emotional response that helps protect the body from harmful substances such as germs and toxins. Fear is usually how we respond to external threats, but disgust functions to keep unsafe substances out of the body.[12] In contamination-focused OCD or health anxiety, this system can become overly sensitive. The body continues to signal that something is unsafe or unclean even after washing, checking, or reassurance. This helps explain why disgust can feel so powerful and persistent, even when no real contamination exists.

## Body Dysmorphia and Muscle Dysmorphia

Body dysmorphic disorder (BDD) is characterized by an excessive preoccupation with a perceived or minor defect in appearance that causes significant distress or impairment. Common symptoms include repetitive checking behaviors, mirror-gazing, comparing one's appearance to others, and reassurance seeking. It affects about 2 percent of people and often co-occurs with conditions like depression, anxiety, eating disorders, and substance use issues.[13] These disorders share a common thread: disruptions in interoception.

Like OCD, body dysmorphia involves intrusive, repetitive thoughts and compulsive behaviors aimed at reducing inner discomfort or uncertainty. The main difference is the focus: Whereas OCD centers on external fears (such as contamination or harm), body dysmorphia's beliefs revolve around the body and self-image.

Muscle dysmorphia (MD) is a subtype of body dysmorphic disorder marked by a preoccupation with not being muscular enough, even in objectively fit individuals. It can lead to compulsive exercise, disordered eating, social withdrawal, and steroid misuse. About 22 percent of men with body dysmorphia meet criteria for MD.[14]

Most research on body dysmorphic disorder has focused on how individuals visually process their appearance, with far less attention to how they perceive and interpret bodily sensations. This gap is important because BDD is a body-focused disorder. Emerging studies suggest that interoception may play a crucial role in both BDD and MD, identifying specific ways altered internal awareness contributes to these conditions.[15]

According to researchers, BDD may involve differences in how the brain interprets bodily signals, especially when there is a mismatch between what someone expects to feel and what their senses detect. A person might genuinely perceive their face as swollen or a feature as not right, even when it appears normal to others. These perceived mismatches can leave parts of the body feeling unsettled, prompting repeated checking, comparing, or avoidance in an understandable effort to find relief—experiences linked to changes in the structure and function of the insula.[16] When the insula's ability to sense and process bodily signals is disrupted, body ownership and self-recognition can weaken, contributing to feelings of detachment, mistrust of the body, and self-objectification—patterns also seen in conditions like anorexia nervosa.[17]

An athlete's goal to gain muscle may seem similar to the pursuit seen in MD, but the two differ in key ways. Athletes typically build muscle to boost performance or meet sport-specific goals. Their training and eating habits are flexible and guided by feedback from their bodies and their coaches. In MD, the motivation to gain muscle is less about performance and more about trying to ease a constant internal sense that the muscles are too small or not right, even when the person is already muscular. Progress may not feel satisfying, reassurance doesn't last, and missing workouts can cause significant distress.

From an interoceptive perspective, MD often involves difficulty sensing and trusting bodily cues. Reduced awareness of hunger, fullness, fatigue, or pain can lead to cycles of overeating when trying to build muscle, extreme restriction when trying to burn fat, or continuing to train despite injury. Eventually, this disconnect from internal signals can foster self-objectification—treating the body as something to control rather than experience—which may increase the risk of extreme behaviors such as steroid use.[18]

Emotional suppression and increased aggression are also more common, reflecting broader challenges with emotional awareness and self-regulation.[19] Overall, research suggests that in both BDD and MD, disruptions in sensing and understanding the body can interfere with how people feel connected to themselves. When the mind–body connection is compromised, body perception can become distorted, emotions harder to regulate, and behaviors more likely to deepen the disconnection.

*Jason, in his early twenties, became focused on building muscle and looking strong. He spent hours lifting weights after long construction shifts, often pushing through pain or injury. Even though he was visibly muscular, he saw himself as "not big enough" and constantly compared his body to other men. Missing a workout made him irritable. Training gave him a sense of control but also reinforced strict ideas about masculinity. When injuries or drinking disrupted his routine, his frustration and anger grew. When he quit training, he replaced exercise with more alcohol.*

*Ava shows patterns typical of body dysmorphia. She spends excessive time obsessing over her appearance—taking and editing many photos of herself, scrutinizing minor flaws in her skin, weight, or facial symmetry, and comparing herself to others. When she feels anxious or rejected, her self-focus intensifies. She cycles through shame, disgust, and anxiety about her body, with brief relief after editing photos, dieting, exercising, or receiving compliments online.*

## Nonsuicidal Self-Injury

Nonsuicidal self-injury (often called NSSI) involves deliberately hurting oneself—such as cutting or hitting—not out of a desire to die, but as a way to manage overwhelming emotions or internal distress. It is most common among teenagers and young adults. Research shows that among adolescents with mental health conditions, the prevalence of NSSI exceeds 40 percent. It frequently occurs alongside conditions like PTSD, depression, OCD, anxiety, eating disorders, and substance use.[20]

The high overlap with other mental health conditions suggests that self-injury is often not an isolated issue but part of a larger struggle with managing intense emotions. Many people who self-injure also experience suicidal thoughts. In one study, more than 82 percent of those who engaged in self-injury had also had suicidal thoughts, highlighting the level of distress they carry.[21]

Although NSSI is not officially classified as an obsessive-compulsive–related disorder, it shares important similarities when viewed through an interoceptive and self-regulation lens. Like checking or skin-picking behaviors, self-injury can function as a repetitive response to emotions that feel intolerable—an attempt to find relief or a sense of calm when distress becomes overwhelming.

### *Interoception and Emotion Regulation in NSSI*

When the body's internal communication system is disrupted, understanding emotions or using body signals to regulate them becomes difficult. For some people, this disruption makes it hard to identify what they are feeling or why. NSSI can be understood as an attempt to cope with this confusion, especially when there's a disconnect between internal sensations and emotional meaning. Emotional overwhelm is one of the main patterns linked to NSSI. Many individuals experience intense states—such as rising tension, agitation, numbness, or emotional overload—that feel confusing or unbearable. When emotions and bodily sensations aren't clearly understood, the resulting internal chaos can be deeply distressing.

Research suggests that individuals with a history of NSSI often struggle to distinguish between bodily sensations and emotions. This can result in an increased focus on bodily cues as they try to make sense of what's happening inside. Self-injury may temporarily lessen this confusion by producing a clear, predictable sensation that feels easier to interpret and control than overwhelming emotions. In other words, NSSI can briefly relieve the tension and uncertainty that arise from emotional and interoceptive confusion.[22]

Self-injury may temporarily resolve this uncertainty in several ways. At a neurobiological level, physical injury triggers the release of neurochemicals that reduce pain and create a short-lived calming or numbing effect.[23] Another possible reason is that self-injury provides a controllable, defined physical sensation that is easier to focus on than the intense emotional distress a person may be experiencing.

*When Ava feels overwhelmed by shame or rejection, she sometimes turns her distress inward. During moments of intense emotional overload, she engages in self-harming behaviors to release tension or manage her internal state. When her usual coping strategies fail, she may overexercise to the point of exhaustion or use physical pain to interrupt her emotional pain.*

### *Disrupted Connection with Self*

One of the most significant interoceptive disruptions linked to self-injury is dissociation, a sense of detachment from one's body or emotions. Up to 86 percent of individuals who experience dissociation also engage in some form of self-harm.[24] Dissociation is a common response to PTSD and childhood trauma; it is the nervous system's way of coping with overwhelming experiences. It can make it harder to stay connected to internal sensations and emotions, creating a sense of separation from the body. When this connection weakens, regulating emotions becomes more difficult, which can increase vulnerability to self-injury.[25]

Research shows that people engage in self-injury for various reasons, including managing trauma-related emotions or intense feelings that are difficult to regulate. For some, NSSI functions as a form of self-punishment tied to emotional dysregulation. For others—particularly those experiencing dissociative symptoms related to PTSD—it may serve as an anti-dissociation strategy. Physical pain can momentarily interrupt numbness or disconnection by restoring sensation,[26] allowing the person to feel more grounded and present in their body. Although the relief is brief, this mechanism helps explain why self-injury becomes a coping strategy when safer ways of grounding or reconnecting with oneself feel out of reach.

Studies indicate that many people who engage in NSSI struggle to trust their bodies. Internal sensations may feel confusing, unreliable, or even unsafe rather than helpful. When this trust is absent, individuals may avoid attending to subtle bodily cues and instead resort to self-injury to create clear, controllable sensations that are easier to interpret. In this way, NSSI can become an alternative method of managing emotions through the body, especially when the body itself feels unfamiliar or distressing. Feeling disconnected from or critical of one's body can also make deliberate self-harm feel more conceivable.[27]

For those who engage in NSSI, simply noticing bodily sensations isn't enough; those sensations must also be interpreted as safe, meaningful, and worth attending to. Rebuilding body trust is often a gradual process, especially when trauma has disrupted that sense of safety and connection. But it is possible when someone feels supported in learning to experience their body as a source of information and stability rather than something to fear.

## How MAIA Domains Can Be Impacted in OCD and Related Disorders

Although OCD and related conditions may appear different on the surface, they share a common pattern of altered interoceptive processing. These are some of the ways MAIA domains can be affected.

**Trust.** This domain is deeply impacted in OCD and related disorders. Bodily sensations are often viewed not as helpful guides or sources of safety but as threatening or misleading. In OCD, sensations of contamination or internal dirtiness trigger distrust and compulsive cleaning. In body and muscle dysmorphia, internal cues are dismissed as flawed or incorrect, reinforcing distorted self-perception. For those who engage in nonsuicidal self-injury (NSSI), bodily sensations may feel meaningless or unsafe, making harm or dissociation more conceivable. Across these conditions, the body becomes unreliable, or even hostile, weakening the belief that internal experiences can be trusted or used to regulate emotions.

**Not-Distracting.** This domain is also heavily affected, often showing a pattern of increased awareness and avoidance. People may become acutely attuned to uncomfortable bodily sensations—such as tension, a sense that things are not right, or disgust—yet feel unable to tolerate them. Because their capacity to regulate these sensations is reduced, they try to escape or control them through repetitive or self-harming behaviors. Checking, picking, or self-injury can momentarily distract from or release inner discomfort, but these actions ultimately heighten sensitivity to the very sensations they aim to avoid. This cycle underscores the importance of learning to stay with distressing internal cues and feelings without immediately trying to alleviate them.

**Self-Regulation.** This ability is also profoundly disrupted among individuals with OCD or related disorders. They often struggle to use bodily awareness to manage emotions or restore a sense of calm. Instead of relying on internal sensations to guide or soothe themselves, they depend on external behaviors—rituals, checking, excessive exercise, or self-injury—to relieve tension or stress. While these behaviors temporarily reduce discomfort, they ultimately reinforce dependence on compulsive patterns rather than genuine self-soothing, making long-term regulation more challenging.

# 15

# Substance Use and Addiction Disorders

In this chapter, we'll examine research on the connection between interoceptive processes and substance use and addiction disorders. This work also allows me to integrate these findings with my own clinical perspective, which centers on the relationship between trauma and addiction. Much of my professional career has been dedicated to exploring this link.

As both a clinician and educator, I've spent years studying how trauma impacts the nervous system and how these effects increase the likelihood of using substances or behaviors to regulate internal states. The more I learn about interoception and how disruptions in this system affect trauma survivors, the clearer the connection between trauma and addiction becomes.

## The Problem Is the Problem

Substance use and addiction disorders remain major health concerns in North America and worldwide. In 2024, nearly fifty million Americans aged twelve and older experienced a substance use disorder (SUD) in the prior year.[1] While alcohol is the most commonly misused substance, other substances—including cannabis, opioids, and cocaine—also contribute significantly to addiction-related harm.

Beyond SUDs, millions worldwide struggle with behavioral addictions like technology dependence, gambling, gaming, shopping, or pornography. A study conducted during the pandemic found that just over 11 percent of people across forty countries experienced some form of behavioral addiction. These countries represent a broad cross section of the global population, including Brazil, China, India, Mexico, Russia, Spain, the UK, and the USA. Technology-related addictions were the most common: smartphone (30.7 percent), social media (15.1 percent), and internet (10.6 percent) addiction.[2]

Many people do not meet diagnostic criteria for addiction or dependence on substances or behaviors, but still experience serious negative consequences.

This chapter explores patterns of substance use and behavioral addiction along a spectrum—from misuse to diagnosed addiction. Whether the behavior involves a substance or an activity, similar patterns emerge: People resort to numbing, distracting, or mood-altering behaviors to cope with internal distress.

When we focus only on the behavior, it's easy to overlook what lies underneath. Substance use and compulsive behaviors are often treated as the problem, yet they are more accurately understood as signals of deeper pain. Addiction is frequently a response to suffering rather than its cause. While these behaviors can lead to significant consequences, understanding why they develop is crucial.

Misuse often begins as an effort to regulate emotional or physical distress—especially distress rooted in trauma or unresolved experiences. As Gabor Maté has noted, we cannot fully understand addiction without asking what relief a person is seeking.[3] At its core, addiction is an attempt to manage overwhelming emotions and bodily sensations, not a pursuit of pleasure.

Trauma can impair the ability to sense, trust, and interpret internal signals. When this internal guidance system is disrupted, people may feel anxious without knowing why, become overwhelmed by emotions they can't regulate, or turn to substances or behaviors for relief. From this perspective, addiction reflects nervous system dysregulation rather than a lack of willpower. Although trauma is not present in every case, problems with interoception are almost always involved.

## The Link Between Trauma and Addiction

The Adverse Childhood Experiences (ACE) Study highlights that trauma is more common than we often acknowledge. Just as importantly, the study underscores the long-term effects early adversity can have on both mental and physical health. One of its key findings is the strong link between ACEs and SUDs: Individuals with higher ACE scores are significantly more likely to struggle with addiction as adults. Those with four or more ACEs are between four and twelve times more likely to develop an alcohol or drug use disorder than those with no ACEs.[4]

Childhood trauma also contributes to difficulties in self-regulation, impulse control, and stress tolerance. When these capacities are compromised, managing emotional and physical distress becomes more challenging. Consequently, individuals with multiple ACEs are at greater risk of turning to substances or compulsive behaviors to cope with overwhelming emotions and bodily sensations.

Traumatic stress can keep the body's alarm system constantly activated, leaving individuals in a state of heightened vigilance. In this state, even neutral sensations or everyday stressors may feel threatening. Prolonged activation of the stress response makes it hard to feel safe, connected, or internally calm.

For some, this ongoing dysregulation shows up as hyperarousal, including hypervigilance, increased startle response, emotional reactivity, muscle tension, headaches, gastrointestinal discomfort, and sleep disturbance. For others, it appears as hypoarousal, marked by fatigue, emotional numbness, dissociation, and a sense of disconnection from the body or environment. In both cases, substances or compulsive behaviors may be used in attempts to soothe the nervous system when internal states become overwhelming.

## "Coping" Through Mood-Altering, Distraction, Numbing, and Avoidance

When people are overwhelmed by symptoms of unresolved trauma, it's natural and understandable for them to escape into self-medication and distraction. Self-medicating refers to the use of alcohol, unprescribed drugs, or certain behaviors to "treat" painful internal experiences such as unresolved trauma, chronic stress, or mental health challenges. Over time, numbing and distraction can become primary coping strategies. While not exhaustive, the following are some of the many substances and behaviors people may use to escape or dull emotional and physical pain.

Common substances used for distraction or avoidance include alcohol, cannabis, opiates, cocaine, hallucinogens, stimulants, caffeine, and nicotine. Technology can also serve as a coping mechanism through excessive use of social media, gaming, or other digital activities. Other behaviors—such as disordered eating, overworking, compulsive shopping, overexercising, or gambling—may offer temporary relief but ultimately increase distress. Compulsive sexual behaviors, including heavy pornography use, high-risk sexual encounters, or chronic infidelity, can serve a similar function: not as pursuits of pleasure, but as attempts to avoid or soothe internal discomfort.

Research shows that unhealthy coping behaviors tend to cluster in patterns, especially when trauma and disrupted interoception are involved. Multiple addictions often co-occur: In one study, nearly half of participants reported at least one excessive behavior in the previous year—about 30 percent reported one excessive pattern, and 21 percent struggled with two or more addictive patterns involving both substances and compulsive behaviors.[5]

In that study, *excessive* referred to the ongoing use of a substance or behavior that causes problems, such as loss of control, neglect of responsibilities, interpersonal conflict, or direct harm to oneself. Many participants reported overlapping patterns—for example, smoking alongside excessive internet use, gambling, or disordered eating; alcohol use alongside problematic social media use, gaming, or gambling; and marijuana use alongside gaming or gambling.[6]

This clustering matters because it highlights how people often rely on multiple strategies to manage confusing or overwhelming internal signals. Each additional unhealthy pattern further disrupts and impairs the ability to sense and respond to one's inner state. These patterns are not random; they reflect underlying difficulties in how the nervous system detects, interprets, and responds to bodily signals. When interoceptive processing is disrupted, stress, emotions, and cravings can become harder to notice and regulate, making substances or compulsive behaviors feel like easier ways to find relief.

## Interoceptive Disruptions in Addiction

Beyond the disruptions caused by trauma, interoceptive difficulties also play a central role in how addictions form and persist. When a person has trouble accurately sensing, interpreting, or trusting their internal bodily signals, everyday experiences—such as stress, anxiety, hunger, loneliness, fatigue, or even the early stirrings of craving—can register only as vague or unpleasant. Without clear internal cues to guide emotional regulation or decision-making, managing impulses or responding adaptively to distress becomes far more difficult.

When internal signals feel unclear, substances and compulsive behaviors can seem like quick, reliable ways to cope with uncomfortable sensations or emotions that aren't fully understood. In time, however, addictive behaviors can distort interoception even further: Some bodily signals become dulled, while others become hypersensitive, making it increasingly confusing or difficult to tune into the body in a coherent way. This creates a self-perpetuating cycle in which disrupted interoception fuels addiction, and addiction worsens interoceptive dysregulation.

The following section outlines several ways in which altered interoception manifests in addictive processes, offering additional insight into how deeply addiction is intertwined with the body's internal sensing systems.

**Alterations in the insula.** SUDs directly affect the insula, the brain region responsible for processing internal bodily signals. A 2024 study demonstrated that alcohol and cocaine addiction can cause structural changes in the insula, including reduced gray matter volume. These alterations may disrupt interoception, impair craving regulation, and diminish impulse control.[7] Since the insula is the brain's central hub for interoception, dysfunction in this area is closely linked to emotional dysregulation, impulsive or risky decisions, and increased cravings—key factors that contribute to and sustain addiction.[8]

**Impaired emotion regulation.** When people struggle to recognize and manage their emotions, they often turn to substances, online activities, or gambling to escape discomfort. Individuals at risk for problematic internet use frequently have difficulty identifying their feelings, rely more on external cues, and have weaker interoceptive skills, making them more reactive to unpleasant bodily sensations.[9] Problematic online behaviors can also serve as coping strategies for loneliness, stress, or negative emotions, and these patterns are often shaped by early caregiving experiences and attachment styles.[10] Research shows that poor emotion regulation and avoidance of emotional awareness are linked to greater severity in gambling disorder.[11]

**Poor interoceptive skills.** Difficulties noticing, naming, or understanding bodily sensations can make people more likely to react without thinking or rely on addictive behaviors to manage vague or uncomfortable nervous system activation. Conversely, being overly sensitive to internal sensations can also be risky, as heightened awareness may intensify cravings, stress responses, and the likelihood of relapse. Thus, both reduced and heightened interoception can contribute to addiction, but through different pathways.[12]

**Impulsivity.** Cognitive neuroscientist Aleksandra Herman, who studies interoception and impulsivity in addiction, notes that individuals who struggle to recognize or make sense of internal cues—such as tension, discomfort, or craving—are more likely to act impulsively to quickly relieve distress. Impulsivity refers to the tendency to pursue immediate rewards without fully considering consequences and is marked by reduced self-control and difficulty delaying gratification, both of which increase vulnerability to addiction. Substance use can further heighten impulsivity by disrupting brain systems involved in self-regulation and decision-making, reinforcing the cycle of use.[13]

**Alexithymia**. Alexithymia—difficulty recognizing and describing emotions—is common in SUDs and behavioral addictions, including gambling disorder and technology addictions. It is closely linked to poor interoception. When interoceptive abilities are weak, internal states such as tension, arousal, or emotional shifts may feel vague or confusing and can be easily misread or misattributed.[14] For example, someone may feel tense or restless but be unable to label the sensation as stress, making substance use or unhealthy coping behaviors an appealing way to manage discomfort. Alexithymia also contributes to increased risks. In gambling disorders, it is associated with greater severity, riskier behaviors, and poorer decision-making.[15]

**Reduced bodily awareness.** Researchers who study problematic internet use describe a "digitalized self," in which people become increasingly immersed in online environments while growing disconnected from their bodily and emotional cues. This can create a feedback loop in which emotional and physical disconnection drives more compulsive online engagement.[16] Gaming research shows similar patterns: Players often report losing track of time, staying up later than planned, skipping meals, or failing to notice fatigue—signs of diminished bodily awareness. These effects are even stronger when players feel a sense of embodiment, perceiving the avatar's body as their own. Reduced bodily awareness can have real health consequences, ranging from disrupted sleep to ignoring signs of exhaustion.[17]

**Cravings.** Individuals with SUDs who experience intense cravings face a higher risk of ongoing use and relapse. Although the mechanisms behind cravings aren't fully understood, poor interoceptive awareness is thought to contribute in two ways. First, when bodily awareness is low, internal warning signals like stress or early withdrawal symptoms may not be clearly perceived, leading individuals to rely on habits or substances to feel better. Conversely, some people experience internal distress much more vividly, especially during stress or withdrawal. Strong negative emotions or physical discomfort can intensify cravings, particularly when substance use is seen as a way to ease that discomfort.[18]

**Withdrawal symptoms.** Withdrawal from addictive substances can involve significant physical discomfort, including nausea, vomiting, tremors, headaches, sweating, fatigue, and muscle aches. Behavioral addictions can also produce withdrawal-like symptoms, such as irritability and restlessness, even without a substance.

When interoceptive awareness is limited, early signs of withdrawal-related discomfort may go unrecognized or be experienced only as vague anxiety or distress. These internal sensations can quietly build and begin to drive behavior, increasing the urge to seek relief.[19] As discomfort intensifies, individuals may feel less able to cope with what is happening internally, making a return to the substance or behavior more likely. When internal regulation feels inaccessible, external soothing through substances or compulsive behaviors can seem like the only option, painfully reinforcing the very pattern they are trying to change.

**Difficulty in recognizing harm.** Disrupted interoception can also reduce the ability to sense the body's natural warning signals about the harmful effects of substances or compulsive behaviors, making it harder to recognize when use has become unsafe and needs to stop.[20] For example, excessive alcohol consumption can irritate and damage the gastrointestinal lining, contributing to inflammation and discomfort.[21] Over time, these internal signals may become easier to overlook or dismiss. When people are less able to detect or interpret concerning bodily cues, riskier patterns of use are more likely to continue.

**The vicious cycle.** Substance use further hampers interoceptive processing by reducing sensitivity to natural rewards—such as enjoying a good meal, connecting with others, or engaging in a satisfying hobby—while intensifying the body's response to substance-related cues. In other words, the body becomes less responsive to healthy sources of satisfaction and more pulled toward the reward of substance use. Similar patterns appear in behavioral addictions, such as gambling, which also involve disrupted interoceptive processes.[22]

## A Nervous System Perspective on Unhealthy Coping

When we look at the wide range of unhealthy coping behaviors—including different types of addiction and mood-altering behaviors—it can be helpful to view them through a nervous system perspective. Many individuals with a trauma history spend prolonged periods in states of heightened activation or shutdown, or they alternate between the two. Heightened activation indicates sympathetic arousal and the hypervigilance commonly linked to trauma. Shutdown states, on the other hand, are marked by disconnection, numbness, and low energy, often seen in trauma-related hypoarousal. In both states, disruptions in interoceptive processing play a key role. When the body's internal signals feel overwhelming, muted, or confusing, emotional regulation becomes harder, and dysregulation can become self-reinforcing over time.

A pattern I often see among clients with both trauma histories and substance use disorders is difficulty accessing a calm, regulated state. The combination of traumatic experiences and long-term patterns of numbing or self-medicating creates such deep dysregulation that many struggle to recognize—let alone sustain—moments of grounding. For some, the idea of feeling more settled or safe in their bodies is unfamiliar. When relief feels out of reach, self-medicating can become a way to cope with the discomfort of living in chronic activation, shutdown, or the exhausting cycle between the two.

Substance use and other mood-altering behaviors temporarily ease survival states and trauma symptoms driven by dysregulated interoceptive cues. These internal sensations are often intensely uncomfortable, leading people to seek any form of relief. In my work with clients, I've noticed that mood-altering behaviors commonly serve four main goals.

### *Staying Activated in Hyperarousal*

Some individuals with highly activated nervous systems may prefer to stay in a heightened state of alertness and hyperarousal. They might turn to numbing or mood-altering experiences that keep them activated, such as stimulant drugs, excessive caffeine, risky behaviors, intense gaming, or compulsive sexual behavior. For these individuals, hyperarousal can feel more manageable—or more familiar—than the vulnerability of a regulated state they cannot access.

> *While Ava's behaviors may not fully meet criteria for addiction, she shows a compulsive pattern of distraction through overexercising, constant social media use, and seeking validation. Rather than soothing her, these habits stimulate her nervous system and keep her in hyperarousal, chasing reassurance and perfection instead of finding calm. The relief she feels is brief, fueling the cycle and keeping her activated, tense, and disconnected from her body.*

### *Taking a Break from Hyperarousal*

Others living in a highly activated state might seek temporary relief from the constant energy, discomfort, or emotional reactivity associated with sympathetic dominance. They may resort to substances or behaviors that calm the system—such as depressants like alcohol, opioids, or cannabis—or opt for more passive forms of disengagement, like mindless scrolling. These options offer a brief respite from anxiety, anger, or feeling overwhelmed.

> *Catherine drinks to turn off her negative self-talk, allowing her to take a break from her relentlessly high expectations of herself.*
>
> *Cannabis helps Jason dial down his stress response. He sometimes uses alcohol the same way, especially when he's alone. But in social settings, alcohol can have the opposite effect. It lowers his inhibitions, clouds his judgment, and amplifies his emotions, making him more reactive and prone to fight responses. In other words, it can keep him activated and stuck in a stress response.*

### *Staying Shut Down*

Individuals prone to hypoarousal and shutting down—those who feel depressed, disconnected, or chronically avoidant—might use substances or behaviors to sustain that numbed, shut-down state. If hypoarousal feels safer or more familiar, they may choose experiences that reinforce disconnection.

> *David often turns to comfort eating and phone scrolling to soothe uncomfortable feelings. These habits provide temporary relief, but afterward he feels sluggish and more disconnected, which keeps him in a shut-down state rather than helping him re-engage with himself or others.*

### *Escaping Numbness*

On the other hand, some individuals who experience significant disconnection and shutdown engage in mood-altering behaviors to feel something other than numbness. When interoceptive awareness is dulled and emotional experience feels distant or inaccessible, activating substances or behaviors can offer a temporary sense of aliveness. This might include using stimulants (cocaine, methamphetamines), engaging in risky activities, sexual acting out, or gambling—anything that pulls them from shutdown into a more activated state.

> *Marcus has felt shut down for months—sleeping long hours, avoiding friends, and moving through life in a fog. Most days, he feels nothing at all. On weekends, he uses stimulants to break through the numbness;*

*the rush briefly makes him feel energized and present. The crash afterward leaves him even more depleted, but the short-lived excitement becomes something he begins to chase.*

## How MAIA Domains Can Be Impacted in Addiction

Although there is considerable variation in interoceptive processes across different types of addiction, some aspects of the MAIA appear to be especially affected in addiction disorders.

**Not-Distracting.** The ability not to distract from uncomfortable sensations and experiences is limited for those with patterns of addiction. People may distract themselves from overwhelming emotions, trauma symptoms, or the early discomfort of craving, hoping the feeling will pass. But when the body's signals are ignored rather than acknowledged, distress often builds up beneath the surface. With time, relying on quick escapes from what feels unbearable inside becomes a contributing factor to addiction.

**Noticing.** This domain is often disrupted in addiction, especially when trauma has played a role. When the nervous system is overwhelmed or shut down, bodily sensations can feel faint, confusing, or too intense to notice. Many people with addiction struggle to detect what's happening inside their bodies—skipping meals, pushing through exhaustion, or losing hours online without noticing their sensations. When early signals are missed, cravings or withdrawal can intensify before being recognized. Reduced awareness of internal cues makes self-regulation more difficult, and the body's messages are more easily overlooked.

**Self-Regulation.** A lack of self-regulation skills is common in addiction disorders. When internal signals are difficult to read or trust, it becomes hard to soothe the body or find a sense of safety from within. Trauma can worsen this, making stress feel intense or unmanageable. Without clear interoceptive cues to guide calming and recovery, people may turn to substances or compulsive behaviors for quick relief. Eventually, this dependence increases, and the body struggles more to regulate emotions or stress on its own.

# 16

# Disordered Eating

Eating disorders develop from a mix of biological, emotional, social, and environmental factors. Genetics, brain chemistry, or pressures from activities such as athletics, modeling, or dance can increase risk, while stress, trauma, and major life changes often lead people to use food or body control as coping mechanisms. Cultural ideals about thinness, health, and appearance add extra pressure, and for many people, food becomes increasingly tied to comfort or coping rather than nourishment.

It's also helpful to distinguish between clinical eating disorders—which involve ongoing patterns of restrictive eating, bingeing, purging, or body-image concerns that significantly affect health and daily life—and disordered eating, which includes harmful habits like chronic dieting or emotional eating that may not meet diagnostic criteria but still cause real distress. Both require care, compassion, and understanding.

While many factors contribute to these struggles, this chapter focuses specifically on how interoception influences and maintains disordered eating behaviors. This view goes beyond ideas of willpower or surface behaviors and highlights challenges in the mind–body connection that often underlie eating-related issues. When hunger, fullness, or emotional cues feel confusing or untrustworthy, people may rely on rules, restriction, bingeing, or compensatory behaviors to feel more in control. Over time, these coping strategies can become self-reinforcing: Discomfort triggers eating behaviors, which then create more discomfort and further disconnection from the body.

Globally, eating disorders impact a significant portion of the population, with lifetime prevalence estimates ranging from 0.74 percent to 2.2 percent in males and 2.58 percent to 8.4 percent in females.[1] Research from another extensive global review indicates that disordered eating behaviors are common among children and adolescents, affecting more than 22 percent of young people worldwide. While not all of these cases meet full diagnostic criteria for an eating disorder, they still reflect a widespread risk among youth.[2]

This chapter examines the spectrum of disordered eating patterns—including anorexia nervosa, bulimia nervosa, binge eating, purging behaviors, and binge eating related to obesity—through the lens of disrupted interoceptive processes. Across this spectrum, a common theme emerges: difficulties sensing, interpreting, trusting, or soothing internal experience. Behaviors such as restricting, bingeing, purging, or overeating often develop as attempts to manage internal discomfort or regulate emotion.

When viewed interoceptively, disordered eating appears less as a set of isolated diagnoses and more as a continuum of disrupted mind–body communication. From this perspective, it becomes clearer how trauma, chronic stress, and insecure attachment can interfere with the ability to sense and trust bodily cues. Interoception offers a useful framework for understanding how confidence in bodily sensations develops or deteriorates, how internal and external cues influence eating behaviors, how hunger and fullness are interpreted, and how predictive processes shape these patterns in time.

## Impacts of Trauma and Insecure Attachment

Research consistently shows a strong connection between trauma and eating disorders. About one in four people with an eating disorder also meet criteria for PTSD.[3] It's not only a history of trauma but also ongoing symptoms, such as intrusive memories, hyperarousal, and emotional numbing, that most strongly shape disordered eating patterns.[4] Individuals with both trauma and an eating disorder often struggle more deeply with mood, anxiety, and self-worth than those with an eating disorder alone.[5]

Trauma can affect how a person sees themselves and their body. Feelings of shame, self-blame, and defectiveness can feed into perfectionism, strict control, and an intense focus on weight and shape.[6] From an interoceptive perspective, trauma disrupts the ability to interpret internal signals—hunger, fullness, and emotional cues may feel confusing, overwhelming, or unreliable. As a result, eating disorder behaviors can act as coping mechanisms: restricting or purging to calm distress, or binge eating to break through numbness. These patterns often mirror trauma's fluctuations between hyperarousal and hypoarousal.

When bodily sensations feel unsafe or unclear, the body can become a place where emotional pain is acted out. Restriction, purging, exercise, or bingeing may serve as ways to manage internal chaos or to feel something when emotions are muted. Early relational trauma—such as insecure attachment and adverse childhood experiences—may further weaken interoceptive trust, making it harder to sense, soothe, and respond to internal experience.[7] In the long term, this disconnection can maintain painful cycles, with the eating disorder functioning not as vanity or choice but as a means of surviving overwhelming internal states.

> *Ava's trauma significantly influences her strict control over her body. Restricting food and overexercising help her feel in control when emotions become too much, and her intense focus on appearance shows a wounded sense of self-worth. Ava copes through her body rather than listening to it. For her, these behaviors aren't about ego—they are ways to manage distress and calm internal chaos.*

Research shows that difficulties trusting and understanding bodily signals play a major role in how insecure attachment contributes to eating disorders, including anorexia nervosa. The lack of confidence in internal cues, such as hunger, fullness, or emotional signals, was so significant that it explained nearly half of the core symptoms of anorexia.[8] For example, hunger signals may seem confusing or unreliable, leading someone to rely less on bodily cues and more on external rules, schedules, or calorie counting to determine when to eat. Alternatively, a feeling of fullness after a meal may seem overwhelming or threatening, causing someone to stop eating early or avoid food to escape those sensations.

When interoceptive development is interrupted by attachment wounds or inconsistent caregiving, hunger and emotional signals may become confusing, and insecure attachment can further erode confidence in these cues. Without a trustworthy inner guide, people may seek reassurance externally—through appearance, control of food or exercise, or external approval. With time, the more someone relies on outside validation, the more disconnected they become from their inner world, which increases the anxiety and body-focused distress seen in restricting types of disordered eating.[9]

## Interoceptive Challenges in Disordered Eating

There are several additional interoceptive patterns that influence disordered eating. The following are some factors that contribute to the complex ways in which interoceptive processes shape eating behaviors.

### *Emotional Dysregulation*

Impaired interoceptive awareness makes internal sensations confusing or difficult to trust. Emotional arousal may be mistaken for hunger or fullness, or bodily sensations may feel overwhelming and hard to interpret. This confusion between emotion and bodily states can complicate regulation, and food-related behaviors often become coping strategies—eating to soothe anxiety or restricting intake when sensations feel uncomfortable or threatening. In this way, disordered eating provides temporary relief from distress while reinforcing patterns that maintain symptoms.[10]

Within this context, behaviors like restriction, bingeing, or purging often act as responses to emotional overload. Although these strategies may offer short-term control or relief, they tend to increase emotional avoidance and further diminish trust in the body. When internal states feel intense or unsafe and healthier regulation strategies are unavailable, severe food restriction may help quiet internal chaos, highlighting the strong connection between interoception, emotion regulation, and eating behaviors.[11]

*After a draining day, Lauren comes home tense and exhausted, unsure whether the tight feeling in her stomach is hunger, fatigue, or stress. Too tired to cook, she reaches for her comfort foods—chips and ice cream—one of the ways she copes when overwhelmed. The relief is brief, soon replaced by tension and guilt for eating more than she intended. In these moments, food offers a temporary escape from emotional overload rather than true hunger, reinforcing disconnection and self-criticism.*

## *Hunger and Fullness Cues*

Interoception plays a vital role in regulating eating behavior by helping us recognize when we are hungry, when we have eaten enough, and when we are satisfied. Clear signals guide us toward balanced, healthy eating. However, when interoceptive communication is disrupted, the brain may misinterpret or miss bodily cues, leading to confusion between physical hunger and emotional needs. Such disruptions are increasingly seen as a key feature of disordered eating.

For instance, in anorexia nervosa, hunger and fullness signals are often altered. People with anorexia usually show reduced sensitivity to hunger and heightened sensitivity to fullness, even when their bodies still need nourishment. This suggests that their brains may be misreading internal cues about when to eat and when to stop. Conversely, individuals with bulimia and binge-eating disorder often experience blunted fullness responses and have difficulty distinguishing between hunger and emotional cues.[12]

## *Impact of External Cues on Disordered Eating*

Another study offers a helpful way to understand the two bodily systems that influence eating habits; both generate interoceptive cues. The first is *homeostatic control*, which regulates hunger and fullness. The second is *hedonic control*, the pleasure-and-reward system that creates the sense of enjoyment we get from food. Ideally, these systems work together: Interoception conveys the body's biological need for nourishment and the satisfaction that comes with eating, while external cues—taste, smell, and other environmental inputs—enhance the experience. When these systems fall out of balance, eating may become guided more by external factors than by internal ones.[13]

For example, when someone has a reduced ability to recognize when they are full, the sensory appeal of food may take on a stronger role, making overeating more likely. Individuals with obesity often have difficulty recognizing hunger and fullness cues and show heightened responsiveness to sight, smell, and other environmental stimuli—a pattern that, in turn, leads to overeating.[14]

Highly processed, palatable foods are intentionally engineered to stimulate cravings and activate the brain's reward pathways. People with disordered eating are particularly vulnerable to these cues because they often struggle to accurately sense hunger, fullness, or satisfaction. This combination makes these foods especially appealing and difficult to stop eating even when full. When interoceptive awareness and reward regulation are impaired, eating becomes driven more by craving and external stimulation than by genuine hunger, further contributing to patterns of disordered eating.

Beyond food cues, social and cultural messages also influence how people relate to their bodies. Research shows that body dissatisfaction and internalizing appearance standards are strong predictors of eating disorder symptoms. A key factor is self-objectification, the tendency to view the body from an outside perspective and judge it based on appearance. When this becomes the focus, visual cues begin to feel more reliable than internal sensations, making it easier for self-worth to hinge on how the body looks rather than how it feels and functions. This disconnection gradually erodes body trust, skews perception, and intensifies disordered eating behaviors.[15]

These pressures do not affect everyone equally. Social media amplifies them, especially for adolescents and young adults. Gender plays a significant role: Girls and young women are bombarded with content idealizing thinness, flawless skin, and beauty routines, while boys and young men increasingly encounter messages equating worth with muscularity, low body fat, and strength. Platforms often elevate white, Eurocentric beauty standards—lighter skin, certain facial features, and specific body shapes. Youth of color may feel pressure to adjust their appearance through filters, grooming, or dieting, or may experience tension between mainstream ideals and cultural norms in their own communities. Instead of fostering genuine health, these expectations deepen disconnection from a true sense of self.

## Predictive Processing

Predictive processing theory offers a valuable framework for understanding how disordered eating develops and persists. It proposes that the brain continually compares what it expects to sense with what it actually perceives, updating its internal model when a mismatch occurs. In eating disorders, this process can become imbalanced, particularly in how the brain interprets interoceptive cues. When signals such as hunger, fullness, or emotional states feel vague or unreliable, the brain may assign less weight to these internal cues and rely more heavily on its expectations, turning instead to external cues like appearance or social standards. This reflects an imbalance in how predictions and sensory signals are weighted.[16]

In anorexia nervosa, this imbalance causes bodily sensations like hunger or fatigue to lose their impact, while rigid beliefs and visual impressions take precedence. The brain gives too much weight to its predictions (I'm still too big) and too little to incoming sensory evidence, even when that evidence clearly contradicts those beliefs. This dynamic results in a distorted, persistent body image and ongoing restrictive eating behaviors.

Across eating disorders, predictive processing highlights a common theme: The brain struggles to integrate real bodily signals with its own expectations. This breakdown in prediction and perception helps explain why distorted body image, emotional distress, and maladaptive eating patterns endure even when confronted with clear physical evidence to the contrary.

## How MAIA Domains Can Be Impacted in Disordered Eating

Here are some of the ways disordered eating patterns interact with the MAIA domains:

**Trust.** This domain reflects a sense of safety and confidence in one's bodily sensations. When someone trusts their body, they can use hunger, fullness, and emotional cues as guides rather than relying on strict rules or external approval. For example, a person with strong body trust might notice they're getting full and comfortably stop eating, believing their body knows what it needs. Someone with low body trust, however, may experience hunger or fullness as confusing or even threatening—hunger might feel like failure or loss of control—leading them to ignore or suppress these cues. Over time, this distrust can raise anxiety and further distance them from their internal experience. Research suggests that body trust may be one of the most important interoceptive skills linked to eating disorders,[17] underscoring its central role in emotional safety and self-regulation around food.

**Not-Worrying.** This domain reflects the ability to experience sensations like fullness, hunger, or tension without reacting with fear or anxiety. Someone stronger in this area might notice fullness after a meal and simply understand it as part of digestion. In contrast, those who worry about bodily sensations may interpret them as threatening—hunger can spark anxiety, and fullness may bring shame or fear of weight gain. When ordinary sensations feel unsafe, people often respond with rigid control, avoidance, or constant monitoring, reinforcing disordered eating patterns and deepening the disconnect from internal cues. Emotional arousal—such as anxiety, sadness, or even excitement—may also be experienced as overwhelming bodily discomfort. In these moments, disordered eating can become a way to escape or quiet sensations that feel too intense to sit with.

**Body Listening.** This domain involves tuning into bodily sensations for guidance and insight. In disordered eating, this capacity is often disrupted. Hunger, fullness, fatigue, and emotional cues may be ignored, mistrusted, or overridden in favor of rigid rules or external guidance about food and body shape. Interestingly, research shows that higher body-listening scores can be maladaptive in some disordered eating patterns.[18] For people who struggle with body trust or feel dissatisfied with their bodies, tuning inward may shift into hypervigilance rather than gentle awareness. Instead of helping them understand their needs, this heightened monitoring can increase anxiety and self-criticism, turning ordinary sensations—like fullness or muscle tension—into sources of worry, guilt, or urges to restrict. In this way, trying to "listen" to the body too closely can paradoxically intensify discomfort and deepen preoccupation with bodily cues.

# 17

# Neurodivergent Conditions

Autism and ADHD are neurodevelopmental conditions often grouped under the broader term *neurodivergence*, which describes differences in brain function and information processing that influence how individuals think, feel, and experience the world. Although they are clinically classified as disorders, many people and researchers see them as natural variations in attention, perception, and sensory processing rather than as deficits. Both perspectives offer value: The medical model supports access to diagnosis, treatment, and accommodations, while the neurodiversity paradigm emphasizes strengths and the importance of accepting different ways of being. Together, they provide a more balanced understanding that recognizes both challenges and the abilities and contributions of neurodivergent individuals.

Growing research on interoception has opened new avenues for understanding neurodivergence. Both autism and ADHD are increasingly linked to alterations in interoceptive processing, which is not surprising given how often individuals with these conditions experience symptoms directly tied to internal sensing. Sensory processing differences are common in neurodivergence: Some people show heightened reactivity to sensory cues, while others display a diminished capacity to identify or interpret them. Challenges in emotional regulation, attention, and sensory processing also frequently overlap with interoceptive disruptions.

This chapter examines interoceptive patterns, including sensitivity and the integration of bodily cues, that shape the distinct cognitive and emotional profiles observed in autism and ADHD.

## Autism Spectrum Disorder

For over a decade, practitioners have developed interoceptive tools and strategies to support individuals diagnosed with autism spectrum disorder

(ASD). Occupational therapist Kelly Mahler has been at the forefront of this work, well before the connection between interoceptive disruptions and mental health challenges became widely recognized. In 2015, she published *Interoception: The Eighth Sensory System*,[1] which explains interoception and offers practical tools to enhance emotional regulation and self-awareness. Her work also emphasizes how interoceptive challenges uniquely affect autistic people and those with related conditions. Since then, Mahler has continued to educate, advocate, and expand understanding of interoceptive differences, helping professionals and caregivers better support those on the autism spectrum. I encourage readers to explore more of her work to better understand the connections between neurodivergence and interoception.

Current research highlights a significant, though complex, relationship between interoceptive processes and ASD. Many autistic individuals experience difficulties with sensory processing and emotional regulation, both of which are closely tied to interoception. Research exploring interoception in ASD highlights key ways internal signals may be experienced and understood.

### *Interoceptive Differences Common in Autism*

Research shows that people with ASD often have trouble sensing and understanding internal body signals, including hunger, thirst, or toileting cues. They are also frequently sensitive to noise or tactile input. Saray Bonete and colleagues identify three primary patterns of interoceptive difficulty characteristic of ASD. These patterns are similar to interoceptive disruptions seen in other mental health conditions.[2]

#### INTEROCEPTIVE HYPOSENSITIVITY

- Low awareness of internal signals related to bodily functions or emotions.
- Sensations are often noticed only when they become intense—for example, not recognizing hunger cues until feeling extremely hungry.

#### INTEROCEPTIVE HYPERSENSITIVITY

- Overly intense or rapid awareness of internal sensations.
- The person may feel many bodily signals at once or too intensely, making it hard to focus on which cues matter most.

POOR INTEROCEPTIVE DISCRIMINATION

- Internal sensations are felt but experienced as vague or confusing.
- The person struggles to identify or describe what they are sensing because the meaning of the sensation is unclear.

Other research on interoceptive abilities in ASD also demonstrates the recurring pattern of hyper- and hyposensitivity. The wide variability in how autistic individuals experience interoceptive cues likely reflects the vast spectrum of autism presentations, including differences in overall severity and individual symptoms. Additionally, ASD often co-occurs with intellectual disabilities or alexithymia, both of which may further interfere with interoception.[3]

## *Difficulty in Interpreting and Integrating Bodily States*

A study by researchers in Japan found that autistic adults can often detect individual bodily signals, such as their heartbeat, yet still experience difficulty understanding their internal states. Rather than an inability to notice sensations, the challenge may lie in organizing and interpreting them, especially when multiple signals must be integrated into a meaningful whole, such as hunger, thirst, or fatigue.[4]

For example, thirst may involve a dry mouth, dry lips, fatigue, or headache—subtle cues that need to be brought together and understood. While individual sensations may be noticed, integrating them into a clear sense of what the body needs can be more difficult for autistic people. A similar pattern may apply to emotional experience, which also depends on combining multiple bodily signals. In this way, the difficulty is not a lack of bodily awareness but a challenge in making sense of internal signals as a coherent whole.

## *ASD, Interoception, and Emotion Regulation*

Interoceptive processes play an essential role in emotional awareness and regulation. These capacities are often impacted in people with ASD, who may find it challenging to connect bodily sensations with emotions. One reason for this is hyposensitivity: A reduced ability to perceive the interoceptive cues generated by emotions can make those emotions harder to identify and regulate.

Research highlights the insula's role in emotional processes, particularly in the context of ASD.[5] As discussed earlier, the insula helps link bodily signals with emotional meaning and plays a key role in experiencing and interpreting emotion-based sensations. In ASD, the insula often shows atypical function or connectivity, which may contribute to difficulties in the early recognition and understanding of emotional cues. When interoceptive skills are diminished, it impacts the ability to recognize challenging emotions early and to use regulation skills before those emotions become overwhelming.

Another factor contributing to emotion-regulation challenges in ASD is the high co-occurrence of alexithymia—difficulty identifying, processing, and describing emotions and bodily sensations. Research suggests that the emotional difficulties often attributed to autism may in fact stem from co-occurring alexithymia.[6] People with alexithymia tend to have less typical emotional awareness, which can make regulation more challenging. The study also emphasizes the role of interoception, noting that both alexithymia and differences in sensing internal bodily cues are linked to brain regions like the insula, which helps connect body signals to emotional meaning. Viewing alexithymia as related to but distinct from autism helps explain why emotional experiences vary so widely among autistic individuals.

A study in this area further underscores the value of more tailored support: Strengthening body awareness and emotional language may improve emotional understanding and social connection, particularly for autistic individuals who also experience alexithymia.[7]

## Attention Deficit Hyperactivity Disorder

Attention deficit hyperactivity disorder (ADHD) affects approximately 5 to 7 percent of children and teens and 3 to 5 percent of adults worldwide.[8] It typically begins in childhood and often continues into adulthood. The primary symptoms include difficulties with focus and attention, impulsivity, and hyperactivity. People with ADHD often describe losing track of time or forgetting tasks, even ones they truly care about. They may speak or interrupt quickly, not out of disrespect, but because their thoughts feel urgent and fast-moving. Many also experience restlessness or a constant need to tap, fidget, or move to stay engaged or focused.

Diagnosis is based on observed symptoms and self-report, as no biological or medical test currently exists to identify ADHD. Symptoms vary significantly among individuals, and many factors influence how they develop and present. Diagnosing ADHD in adults is especially challenging because its symptoms frequently overlap with those of other mental health conditions. More than half of adults with ADHD have at least one co-occurring disorder, such as anxiety, depression, substance use disorder, or a personality disorder.[9]

## *Evolving Perspectives on ADHD*

Identifying the causes and contributing factors of ADHD has proven to be challenging because of multiple overlapping approaches. Research has examined numerous influences that are thought to contribute to ADHD, including genetic factors, environmental conditions such as stress and trauma, and differences in brain development and neurobiological systems.[10] Traditionally, ADHD was identified primarily through its core behavioral symptoms: inattention, impulsivity, and hyperactivity. Over time, however, the understanding of ADHD has evolved, and it now incorporates several complementary perspectives, each offering insight into its complexities. The most common include

**A neurodevelopmental perspective.** A widely accepted scientific and clinical view is that disruptions in brain development contribute to ADHD. Brain imaging studies have revealed notable differences in both the structure and function of the brains of people with ADHD, particularly in regions related to motivation, emotion processing, and cognitive skills such as critical thinking and problem-solving.[11]

**An executive-function perspective.** Another well-supported hypothesis emphasizes that ADHD is primarily a deficit in self-regulation and executive functioning rather than a simple deficit of attention. Executive functions are a set of cognitive skills, including planning, critical thinking, time management, and organization. This model suggests that abnormalities in the brain give rise to these impairments and, in turn, to ADHD symptoms.[12]

**A nervous system dysregulation perspective.** This model interprets ADHD-related behaviors as signs of a nervous system with reduced capacity to regulate stress responses. When the nervous system is dysregulated, symptoms such as impulsivity and poor emotional regulation become more pronounced.[13]

**A trauma-informed perspective.** Research consistently shows significant overlap between trauma and ADHD. Numerous studies indicate that childhood trauma, adverse childhood experiences, and chronic stress can contribute to the development of ADHD symptoms. Children exposed to traumatic events or high levels of stress are more likely to exhibit ADHD-related behaviors.[14] Greater exposure to childhood adversity is also linked to more severe symptoms, particularly impulsivity.[15]

## *Dysregulation: A Core Feature of ADHD*

Our understanding of ADHD increasingly highlights it as a condition of dysregulation, meaning the brain has difficulty maintaining balance and control over key functions such as attention and behavioral responses. Even the name *attention deficit hyperactivity disorder* reflects this point, though individuals with ADHD commonly experience disruptions across multiple areas of functioning. Emotional dysregulation, for example, is now widely recognized as a common feature of ADHD, with high irritability, anger, and ineffective emotion regulation strategies often appearing as its key indicators.[16]

Sensory dysregulation is another core feature of ADHD and contributes to varied reactions to sensory input, including sound, touch, and visual stimuli. From an interoceptive standpoint, sensory input also includes internal bodily signals such as hunger, thirst, or pain. According to researchers, sensory dysregulation includes four patterns:[17]

**Hypersensitivity or sensory overresponsivity.** Exaggerated or prolonged reactions to sensory input. Sensory signals, including interoceptive cues, are amplified and may produce strong emotional responses.

**Hyposensitivity or sensory underresponsivity.** Diminished or delayed reactions that can resemble indifference to environmental stimuli. Hyposensitivity may manifest as a high pain threshold, gripping too tightly, or unawareness of hunger or thirst cues.

**Sensory-seeking behavior.** A craving for sensory input that may present as increased movement, noisemaking, or high-risk behaviors.

**Sensory avoidance.** Withdrawal from stimulation due to low tolerance for sensory input. Examples include relying on noise-canceling headphones or avoiding certain clothing textures.

Research shows that children with significant sensory dysregulation often experience greater-than-expected difficulties in physical, emotional, social, and academic situations.[18] These findings underscore the considerable impact of sensory processing challenges on individuals with ADHD, shaping not only behavior but also how they perceive, interpret, respond to, and navigate their environments in daily life.

Several ADHD symptoms can also be understood as forms of nervous system dysregulation. Sensory dysregulation can be considered part of this broader pattern. One study identified disruptions in the autonomic nervous system seen in both ADHD and PTSD, including impulsivity, excessive motor activity, and an exaggerated startle response—symptoms associated with hyperarousal in PTSD.[19]

Another study looked at dissociative experiences in people with ADHD who also had a history of trauma. They found strong links among ADHD, emotional abuse and neglect, PTSD symptoms, and dissociation—a common hypoarousal response that can develop after trauma. The researchers suggested that dissociative symptoms may contribute to attention difficulties in ADHD.[20] Since childhood trauma increases the risk of ADHD,[21] it's possible that some aspects of nervous system dysregulation in ADHD are influenced by trauma or chronic stress. There is more on this below.

Emotional, sensory, and nervous system dysregulation are closely linked, and this relationship greatly shapes how ADHD manifests in everyday life. When stress or trauma shape the nervous system, staying regulated becomes even more challenging. Persistent hyperarousal or hypoarousal can increase sensory sensitivity, making everyday sounds, textures, or demands feel either overwhelming or barely noticeable.[22] These sensory shifts often affect emotional responses, leading to irritability, frustration, or rapid emotional changes. Over time, these forms of dysregulation can reinforce one another, creating a cycle that makes focus, impulse control, and overall stability harder to sustain.

## *The Trauma–ADHD Connection*

From an interoceptive perspective, it is essential to summarize the link between trauma and ADHD symptoms. Research clearly establishes this connection, as demonstrated in a 2023 review of numerous ADHD studies. The review found that children with no adverse childhood experiences (ACEs) were far less likely to develop ADHD, whereas both the likelihood and severity of ADHD symptoms increased with the number of ACEs a child experienced. Children with four or more ACEs had the highest odds of receiving an ADHD diagnosis and of presenting with moderate to severe symptoms. The study also observed that specific adversities—such as socioeconomic hardship, parental divorce, parental mental illness, and neighborhood violence—significantly increase the likelihood of developing ADHD.[23]

This link between trauma and ADHD risk suggests that early exposure to stress and adversity can shape the developing brain in ways that affect regulation, emotion, and behavior. Numerous studies show that childhood trauma and stress disrupt both the structure and function of brain circuits involved in executive function, attention regulation, and emotion regulation.[24] When these vital circuits are altered by trauma, they can contribute to additional symptoms often seen in ADHD, including increased reactivity, impulsivity, emotional volatility, irritability, hyperactivity, learning difficulties, heightened startle responses, and dissociation. This overlap is crucial to consider when diagnosing or treating ADHD.

When I first began my clinical practice, I worked in a trauma-treatment program for children and teens, where ADHD diagnoses were not uncommon. We saw that when trauma symptoms were addressed and children received support to heal from adverse experiences, many of their ADHD symptoms diminished or disappeared. This is not to say that ADHD is simply unrecognized trauma; rather, it underscores the importance of identifying and treating any underlying nervous system dysregulation resulting from childhood trauma or chronic stressors. When the contributions of trauma are overlooked in diagnosing ADHD, treatment may focus solely on managing symptoms rather than addressing the underlying causes.

## How MAIA Domains Can Be Impacted in Autism and ADHD

Given the wide range of dysregulation seen in autism and ADHD—whether it be emotional, nervous system, or sensory—it is clear that interoceptive processes are also involved, even though these patterns may express themselves differently. Using the MAIA framework, we can see how specific domains may be affected in each condition. And regardless of whether trauma contributes to ADHD symptoms or whether interoceptive disruptions cause or result from them, it is vital to consider how interoceptive processes fit into the overall picture of ADHD.

**Attention Regulation.** This domain involves noticing bodily sensations with enough awareness and steadiness to understand what they signal. In autism, shifting attention between internal cues and the external world can be challenging. Some individuals may hyperfocus on a single sensation or thought, while others may lose awareness of their bodies when engaged in external tasks. This imbalance can make it harder to track internal states in real time. In ADHD, attention regulation is a core challenge, which naturally affects interoceptive awareness. Because attention shifts quickly and inconsistently, tuning in to bodily signals can be difficult, and subtle cues may be missed. This reduced connection to internal sensations can disrupt mind–body communication and make it harder to notice emotions or regulation needs before they intensify.

**Emotional Awareness.** Individuals with ASD often show reduced emotional awareness. They may notice physical sensations—such as a tight chest or a racing heart—but struggle to connect them to specific emotions. Co-occurring alexithymia is common and can further complicate identifying and expressing feelings, affecting emotional regulation and the ability to read social cues. In ADHD, emotional awareness is also frequently disrupted, but often for different reasons. Difficulty sustaining attention to bodily cues in the moment can mean that internal sensations are missed, making it harder to recognize emotions before they escalate. High rates of alexithymia in ADHD further contribute to emotional misinterpretation and quick emotional reactivity.

**Self-Regulation.** For autistic individuals, self-regulation becomes harder when interoceptive cues are faint, confusing, or go unnoticed. Without recognizing early signs of discomfort or emotional activation, it is more difficult to intervene before feelings intensify, contributing to the emotional dysregulation often seen in ASD. In ADHD, self-regulation challenges frequently stem from issues with attention and emotional awareness. When internal signals are missed or recognized too late, it becomes harder to access strategies that soothe, slow down, or restore balance. This can lead to quick escalations, trouble calming the nervous system, and difficulties maintaining emotional stability during stress.

# 18

# Physical Health

One clear theme throughout this book is that interoception and mental health are deeply intertwined. The brain and body share networks that constantly exchange information, and when this communication becomes disrupted, it can contribute to emotional distress and mental health challenges. But the effects of disrupted interoception extend beyond emotional or psychological symptoms—physical health is also profoundly connected to interoceptive processes. When interoception functions well, it helps regulate bodily systems to maintain health. Conversely, altered interoception can be both a cause and a consequence of health problems, creating a cycle that links physical and mental suffering.

Physical and mental health shape each other, and this influence runs in both directions. Chronic physical illnesses such as diabetes, heart disease, and autoimmune conditions increase the risk of depression and anxiety. Meanwhile, untreated mental health issues can worsen physical health, whether through poor sleep, reduced motivation for self-care, or medication side effects that introduce additional strain.

Research shows that alterations in nearly all bodily systems are linked to mental health conditions,[1] with interoception serving as the bridge between mind and body. Conditions like cardiovascular disease, immune dysfunction, and long COVID often coincide with depression, fatigue, and cognitive fog—showing how disrupted internal signaling affects both physical and emotional states. Similarly, people with heart disease experience depression at nearly three times the rate of those without it, and individuals with PTSD face higher risks of high blood pressure and stroke.[2]

Stress—especially when it is chronic or traumatic—is a significant disruptor of brain–body communication. While short-term stress helps the body respond to immediate challenges, long-term stress keeps systems such as the cardiovascular, immune, and digestive systems on high alert. This prolonged overactivation blurs the body's internal signals, fueling inflammation, pain, and mood disturbances. The ACE Study clearly shows that early trauma can have lifelong effects on physical and mental health.[3]

When stress, illness, or trauma interferes with interoception, mind–body communication is altered, leading to heightened anxiety, blunted emotions, chronic pain, or more significant health symptoms. Understanding these shared pathways offers a powerful way to view mental and physical health not as separate domains but as distinct interconnected expressions of the same underlying system. A deeper exploration of chronic pain, irritable bowel syndrome, and migraines can illustrate how the interlinked systems of interoception, mental health, emotions, and physical health continuously interact and affect one another.

## Chronic Pain

In the United States, chronic pain affects more people than diabetes, heart disease, cancer, and stroke combined.[4] It has become one of the most widespread and challenging health issues. Chronic pain takes many forms, including migraines, irritable bowel syndrome, chronic back pain, fibromyalgia, and pain that persists after an injury. There are also multiple approaches to understanding chronic pain, from traditional medical models to the biopsychosocial model and models that emphasize the role of the brain or nervous system. As the science of interoception advances, awareness of the link between chronic pain and interoceptive processes continues to grow. Pain is not just a sensory experience; it is deeply tied to how the brain interprets and processes internal sensation cues, which in turn shape interoceptive processes.

From an interoceptive standpoint, chronic pain stems not only from changes in the body and nervous system but also from how the brain perceives and responds to those signals. When patterns like hypervigilance or central sensitization develop, bodily sensations can become amplified, leading to more intense and lasting pain. This demonstrates a two-way interaction between body and brain: The body may send strong or confusing signals upward, while emotions, memories, and attention influence how those sensations are experienced. When this system becomes tuned to danger or threat, the nervous system remains on high alert, keeping pain active. Effective treatment often involves helping the brain and body communicate more accurately and safely, reducing fear-based responses and creating space for relief.

## *Maladaptive Body Awareness*

A common theme across many health and mental health conditions is maladaptive bodily awareness. Instead of interoceptive cues offering useful information that guides healthy behavior, certain physical sensations may be misinterpreted, overly focused on, or ignored. The interoceptive disruptions seen in chronic pain frequently appear in mental health issues as well. Researchers have identified several distinct yet overlapping concepts related to chronic pain.

**Hypervigilance.** This refers to an exaggerated alertness to pain-related threats or guarding against potential threats.[5] People with chronic pain may constantly monitor for signs of pain or the possibility of worsening symptoms. This can include scanning for pain signals, avoiding certain activities, struggling to relax, or frequently tracking their pain levels.

**Somatic amplification.** This occurs when physical sensations are perceived as more intense, uncomfortable, or threatening than they actually are. This heightened awareness is often connected to strong emotional reactions and the interpretation of bodily cues as signs of illness or danger. When sensations are viewed through a lens of worry or fear, the nervous system reacts more strongly, further amplifying physical discomfort and creating a cycle of tension, vigilance, and distress.[6] Essentially, the brain sometimes overpredicts potential harm, resulting in stronger physical responses.

For example, someone with chronic back pain may scan their body throughout the day for signs of discomfort. Normal sensations—such as a quick muscle twitch or mild stiffness—can quickly become the focus of attention. Because the brain expects pain, neutral signals may be interpreted as threatening, and the more attention they receive, the stronger they feel. A small cue can then be experienced as sharp or alarming pain. This pattern shows how somatic amplification can intensify sensations and increase pain-related fear and vigilance.

**Pain catastrophizing.** This is a particular thinking pattern in which pain is interpreted as more serious, threatening, or unmanageable than it may actually be. Instead of responding only to the physical sensation, the mind begins to imagine worst-case scenarios, which can increase fear and emotional stress. This worry often leads to avoiding movement or activities to stay "safe," even when those activities may be beneficial. Pain catastrophizing isn't just about the sensation itself—it's about the meaning attached to it. Because our thoughts and feelings influence how we perceive bodily sensations, catastrophizing can significantly contribute to maintaining or worsening chronic pain.

**Misinterpretation of signals.** Research suggests that people living with chronic pain often show a mixed pattern of interoceptive awareness: They notice bodily sensations more easily yet struggle to interpret them accurately. In other words, internal signals become louder but less clear.[7] This can lead to increased worry and a tendency to focus on sensations that feel uncertain or potentially threatening. When body cues are misread, awareness shifts from understanding the body to monitoring for danger. Sensations that might otherwise seem neutral can feel urgent, fueling vigilance and tension. Over time, this pattern can reinforce a cycle of pain, anxiety, and avoidance—creating a feedback loop in which misinterpretation heightens distress and pain rather than easing it.

## *Central Sensitization and Chronic Pain*

Central sensitization (CS) is a condition in which the central nervous system becomes overly responsive to pain signals, increasing the perception of pain so that it feels stronger, more persistent, and sometimes disconnected from actual injury or tissue damage. In this heightened state, even light touch or gentle movement can be painful, and sensations like burning, tingling, or stabbing pain may occur without clear tissue damage.[8] Essentially, the brain and spinal cord become "better at producing pain,"[9] keeping the nervous system on high alert.

Biologically, CS develops when nerve cells in the central nervous system fire more easily, send stronger signals, and lose some of their natural ability to dampen pain. Eventually, new neural patterns form that maintain the pain response even when the body provides only minimal input.[10] Emotional and cognitive factors—such as pain catastrophizing, fear, avoidance, and constant monitoring of symptoms—can further strengthen this cycle, increasing sensitivity and reinforcing the nervous system's threat response.

CS is believed to contribute to conditions such as fibromyalgia, irritable bowel syndrome, chronic fatigue, chronic whiplash, low back pain, and migraines. People with CS often experience more severe pain and may respond less to traditional medical treatments.[11] Overall, CS reminds us that chronic pain is not solely a reflection of physical injury; it is shaped by the ongoing interaction between bodily signals, nervous system sensitivity, and the meanings and emotions attached to those sensations.

## Irritable Bowel Syndrome

Irritable bowel syndrome (IBS) is a common condition affecting an estimated 10 to 20 percent of people worldwide. It is considered a functional rather than a structural disorder, meaning symptoms occur even though the bowel appears normal on medical exams. IBS is characterized by chronic or recurring abdominal discomfort along with changes in bowel habits such as diarrhea, constipation, or a combination of both. Because no clear structural damage is found, IBS is now understood as a disorder involving communication between the gut and the brain.[12]

A growing body of research suggests that interoceptive dysfunction plays a key role in IBS. Many individuals with IBS experience gut sensations—such as fullness, bloating, pressure, or pain—as unusually intense or distressing. Neuroimaging studies support this connection, showing changes in brain regions involved in processing internal bodily signals, including the insula.[13] These interoceptive patterns mirror those seen in other chronic health and mental health conditions. Heightened sensitivity to internal cues, stress, emotional reactivity, and alterations in the gut–brain axis can interact to worsen both physical and emotional symptoms, helping explain why IBS can be persistent and challenging to manage.

### *Visceral Hypersensitivity*

Individuals with IBS are more sensitive to sensations in their digestive system, so normal experiences like bloating, intestinal pressure, or bowel movements can feel unusually painful or uncomfortable. This increased gut sensitivity is a form of somatic amplification focused on the gastrointestinal system, where ordinary internal sensations are perceived as stronger or more distressing than they actually are.

The brain interprets gut messages as more intense or alarming, triggering emotional and behavioral responses such as anxiety, fear of symptom flare-ups, avoidance of certain foods or social settings, and increased bodily vigilance.[14] This hypervigilance gradually reinforces a self-perpetuating cycle of discomfort, stress, and symptom severity.[15]

### *IBS and Stress*

Stress plays a key role in both triggering and worsening IBS symptoms, often increasing pain and overall sensitivity. For many people, this acute discomfort is linked to dysregulation in the autonomic nervous system, making it harder for the body to shift naturally between activation and relaxation.[16] Researchers highlight that stress and trauma can interfere with autonomic regulation—especially the vagus nerve, which supports digestion, pain regulation, and emotional balance. When these pathways are disrupted, the body may remain stuck in a heightened state of stress, creating ongoing physiological strain. This may help explain why individuals with trauma histories are more likely to develop gastrointestinal issues and often report more intense IBS symptoms.[17]

When the sympathetic nervous system remains highly activated—as if the body is stuck in a low-grade fight-or-flight response—it stays tense, alert, and ready to react. In this state, normal digestive processes are diminished, and less energy is available for healthy gut function. With time, stress can aggravate intestinal inflammation, alter digestive secretions, and increase sensitivity within the gut lining.[18]

Many individuals with IBS show this pattern: The stress response system is overactive while vagal tone—the calming pathway that supports rest, digestion, and recovery—is reduced.[19] This imbalance can raise cortisol levels and keep the body in an amplified stress cycle, contributing to abdominal pain, bloating, and irregular bowel habits.[20] Emotional factors such as anxiety, depression, and ongoing life stress frequently intensify symptoms, making the nervous system even more reactive.

Viewed through this lens, IBS is not only a gastrointestinal disorder but also a reflection of how the nervous system adapts to stress over time. When stress or trauma has been part of a person's history, the body can become more alert and sensitive to internal sensations, making discomfort feel more intense and more easily triggered. This helps explain IBS symptoms—such as abdominal pain, bowel irregularity, and emotional reactivity—as the body's response to chronic stress and reduced autonomic regulation within the gut–brain axis.[21] These physiological patterns can eventually reinforce cycles of reactivity and often appear alongside challenges in emotional processing, shaping how individuals notice, interpret, and respond to sensations and feelings within their bodies.

## *Gut–Brain Axis*

When we understand how stress and nervous system dysregulation contribute to IBS, it becomes clear that this condition is more than a digestive problem. It is closely linked to disruptions in the gut–brain axis and how the body sends, receives, and interprets internal signals. Many of the gut–brain functions described in Chapter 5, and their impact on interoceptive awareness, are affected in IBS.

Giuseppe Marano and colleagues reviewed and organized current research to summarize what is now known about IBS, with particular attention to women, who experience the condition at higher rates. They describe IBS as a disorder in which communication between the gut and brain becomes dysregulated. In a healthy system, the gut sends signals to the brain about digestion, fullness, discomfort, and even emotional states, while the brain helps regulate intestinal motility, inflammation, and the balance of gut microbes.[22]

In IBS, this communication shifts. The gut can grow more sensitive to internal sensations (visceral hypersensitivity), meaning that normal digestive activity may feel painful or urgent. Gut dysbiosis, or imbalance in gut bacteria, can worsen this by affecting serotonin levels, immune function, and inflammation. Changes in gut motility, whether things move too quickly, too slowly, or irregularly, also contribute to unpredictable symptoms.[23]

These shifts not only affect the body but also influence how the brain interprets sensory signals from the gut. When interoceptive cues are louder, harder to interpret, or more uncomfortable, people may struggle to understand what their body is trying to communicate, leading to confusion, anxiety, and increased awareness of symptoms. In this way, the work of Marano and colleagues emphasizes IBS as a gut–brain axis disorder where physical, emotional, and sensory processes continually shape each other and where improving symptoms may involve supporting both digestive function and the nervous system's ability to feel safe and regulated.

### *Challenges with Emotion Processing*

Interoception is essential for emotional experience and regulation. Because the gut is one of the body's most signal-rich interoceptive organs, disruptions in gut–brain communication can directly impact how a person perceives and responds to feelings. Research indicates that while people with IBS can feel and generate emotions, they often struggle more with understanding, managing, or expressing them clearly. Emotional tolerance can be especially difficult; when gut sensations become intense or confusing, emotions may feel overwhelming, increasing both physical and emotional distress. Some individuals also find it hard to differentiate and classify their emotions, making it challenging to identify what they are feeling. Without clear emotional signals, regulation becomes more difficult, which can lead to coping strategies like suppression, avoidance, or rumination.[24]

IBS affects far more than digestion. It also influences interoceptive awareness, shaping how internal sensations are perceived and how emotions are processed. When gut signals feel intense or confusing, emotional regulation becomes harder, which can cause symptom flare-ups and reduced well-being. Understanding this connection can be empowering. It highlights that IBS is not only a gut problem but also involves the nervous system and the body's interpretation of internal cues. This perspective opens the door to approaches that support both gut health and emotional regulation, improving overall well-being.

*Lauren's IBS tends to flare during periods of emotional overload. When her gut tightens, she struggles to tell whether she's feeling anxious or experiencing digestive discomfort, leaving her unsure how to respond. Stress worsens her symptoms, and her symptoms increase her stress, creating a reinforcing cycle. She often pushes through or ruminates instead of tuning into what she needs. For Lauren, IBS isn't just physical—it reflects how her nervous system processes emotions, making her highly sensitive to internal signals but not always confident in interpreting them.*

## Migraines

Migraine is a common neurological disorder affecting more than one billion people worldwide. It affects more women than men and is one of the leading causes of disability, contributing to significant personal and economic hardship.[25] It is included in this chapter because it is increasingly understood as a condition closely linked to interoception.

Anyone who has had migraines knows the wide range of bodily sensations involved: intense head pain, nausea, dizziness, and heightened sensitivity to sensory input like sound or smell. Many people also notice subtle early cues that warn of an impending migraine, including mood shifts, brain fog, or visual auras. Beyond these physical sensations, other aspects of interoceptive processing also play an important role. Let's take a closer look.

### *Sensory Hypersensitivity*

A study examined the connection between migraines and sensory hypersensitivity. Most participants reported at least one form of sensory sensitivity, most commonly to light, sound, or smell, and more than 41 percent experienced all three. Individuals with multiple sensitivities also reported more frequent migraine attacks and higher levels of distress. Importantly, these sensory disturbances often appeared *before* the onset of pain, indicating they are not merely side effects of the headache. The study's authors propose that these sensitivities reflect disruptions between the interoceptive and sensory processing systems—specifically, abnormalities in how the brain interprets and integrates bodily signals with external stimuli such as light or noise.[26]

Brain imaging studies show that people with migraines often have nervous systems that react more strongly to sensory input. Everyday light, sound, or movement can feel intensified, as if the brain is closely monitoring incoming signals and responding quickly. Researchers believe this may happen because the brain combines sensory information in a way that allows one stimulus—such as light—to amplify the effects of others, like sound or smell. When communication between brain regions becomes more sensitive or easily triggered, multiple sensory inputs can accumulate, helping to explain why migraines often involve several sensitivities and why the overall experience can feel so overwhelming.[27]

## *Predictive Processing and Migraines*

Another way to understand interoceptive disruptions in migraines is through the predictive processing framework. A study by Akihiro Koreki and colleagues found that the brains of people with migraines often generate strong predictions about bodily sensations, but these predictions are not always accurate.[28] Because the nervous system is trying to protect the body from pain, it may jump to conclusions based on past experiences and interpret normal sensations as warning signs. For example, a mild neck ache might immediately be read as *A migraine is starting*, even if it is simply tension or fatigue. Someone who has been sensitive to light during previous attacks may predict that *Light will make this unbearable*, or assume that *Any screen time will trigger an attack*, even when the current situation is different.

Over time, these overly confident predictions can become rigid and difficult to update, even when new sensory information suggests that things are safe. As prediction errors accumulate, the nervous system may become more reactive and sensitive, contributing to chronic pain and a heightened sense of threat within the body.[29]

The same study also noted that key interoceptive brain regions, including the insula, become more active during migraine attacks.[30] This means that the very areas involved in sensing and interpreting internal bodily signals are also heavily engaged in creating migraine symptoms. In other words, migraines are not just reactions to external triggers but are rooted in altered internal monitoring—a miscommunication in how the brain predicts and manages bodily states. When these prediction systems become imbalanced, sensory cues can feel more intense and threatening, leading to interoceptive confusion, increased sensitivity, and the pain and exhaustion that many people with migraines know too well.

*Hailey's migraines often begin with worry rather than pain. Because she's highly attuned to her body, small sensations—like tension or eye strain—can make her fear that a migraine is coming. She becomes alert and cautious, avoiding triggers and checking for symptoms, which unintentionally reinforces the sense that her body is in danger. In time, this pattern heightens her sensitivity, so even ordinary discomfort can feel threatening and stressful.*

## How MAIA Domains Can Be Impacted in Chronic Pain, IBS, and Migraines

Across chronic pain, irritable bowel syndrome, and migraines, a similar pattern emerges: The way internal bodily signals are sensed and interpreted becomes disrupted. Sensations can feel intense or confusing, and harder to trust or understand. This often leads to worry, increased attention to symptoms, and efforts to avoid discomfort, which can unintentionally heighten both physical and emotional distress. In the long term, the body's signals feel less like helpful guides and more like sources of uncertainty, creating a cycle in which stress and symptoms continually reinforce each other. Several domains of the MAIA are affected in similar ways, though each condition has its own nuances:

**Noticing.** Distressing bodily signals are noticed more intensely across all three disorders, reflecting a state of hyperawareness that isn't always accurate or balanced. In chronic pain, attention naturally gravitates toward areas that hurt. In IBS, even normal sensations like bloating or pressure may be misinterpreted as painful or alarming. In migraines, early cues such as light sensitivity, muscle tension, or nausea are easier to notice and can trigger anticipatory anxiety. Across all three conditions, noticing tends to center on discomfort, making sensations seem larger and more urgent. Instead of helping someone understand what their body needs, this heightened awareness can raise distress and obscure neutral or pleasant sensations that might otherwise provide grounding or comfort.

**Not-Worrying.** Scores in this domain tend to be low, as people with these disorders often respond to bodily sensations with anxiety or worry rather than calmness. In chronic pain, this may look like catastrophizing—seeing pain as a sign of serious injury or worsening symptoms. In IBS, worry focuses on gut sensations and the fear of discomfort or flare-ups. For people with migraines, even small cues like a flicker of light or slight nausea can spark anticipatory anxiety about an oncoming attack. Instead of remaining neutral or informative, sensations quickly become sources of emotional distress or worry, making the body feel unpredictable and unsafe.

**Trust.** Across these conditions, trust in the body is low, which can make internal sensations feel unsafe or unreliable. In chronic pain, the body feels untrustworthy as pain persists without a clear cause, leading to fear and avoidance. In IBS, mistrust often centers on the gut, which can feel unpredictable and disruptive to daily life without warning. For people with migraines, uncertainty about when an attack will occur can create vigilance and even a sense of betrayal toward bodily cues. In all three cases, this loss of trust leads individuals to view their bodies as sources of threat rather than guidance.

# 19

# Interpersonal Connections

Everywhere we look, people seem to be struggling to stay connected—both to themselves and to each other. Many feel more isolated than ever. The pull of phones and technology has replaced many of our relational, face-to-face interactions. At the same time, growing polarization and conflict reflect a deeper sense of disconnection. Because interoception is central to how we relate to ourselves, disruptions in interoception naturally affect how we connect with others.

We have come to understand the many ways altered interoception can manifest: pushing through discomfort, ignoring or doubting the body's signals, struggling to link sensations with emotions, or finding it difficult to regulate them. When we dismiss these signals, we lose access to important information that helps us stay grounded and connected to ourselves. These same patterns often appear in our relationships, shaping how we respond to and communicate with others.

Relationship challenges can take many forms, including increased conflict, trouble expressing emotions, a lack of empathy, or emotional overreactions. These aren't just social struggles; they point to deeper disruptions in how we understand and regulate our inner world. When we lose touch with our body's signals, we also lose the foundation that supports empathy, trust, and healthy boundaries. And just as disrupted interoception can make connection harder, the reverse is also true. Without safe, supportive relationships, one's own sense of balance and regulation becomes more fragile. This can lead to anxiety, depression, avoidance, and emotional dysregulation—patterns that eventually create more distance from ourselves and from others.

Strengthening our connection to interoceptive awareness can improve both mental and physical well-being and deepen our relationships. The reverse is equally true: Safe, supportive relationships help us stay more regulated and connected to ourselves. It's a two-way street—inner awareness supports connection, and connection supports inner awareness.

## Attachment, Co-Regulation, and Interoception

Earlier in the book, we explored how early attachment experiences shape interoceptive awareness. When caregivers respond with warmth and attunement—naming feelings, offering comfort, noticing needs—children learn to understand their internal cues and connect sensations with meaning. Supportive caregiving also teaches the body how to shift from distress to calm, a process called co-regulation. In time, these safe relational experiences build secure attachment, strengthen the capacity for social engagement, and support healthy emotional and interoceptive development.

When care is inconsistent, dismissive, or frightening, this process becomes disrupted. The nervous system shifts toward protection—either into hyperarousal or into shutdown.[1] As a result, children may become less able to notice, interpret, or trust their internal signals. Without a sense of safety, the body remains in a protective survival mode instead of learning to feel and understand itself.

### *Early Relational Experiences Shape Adult Ones*

The connection between attachment, interoception, and co-regulation highlights how deeply early caregiving influences our ability to feel safe, connected, and emotionally regulated in adulthood. Even though humans are wired for connection, experiences like inconsistent attunement or attachment trauma can make it harder to access that sense of safety in adult relationships.

Patterns formed in childhood often continue to shape how we relate, feel, and cope. Someone with an anxious attachment style may remain highly attuned to bodily sensations, sometimes interpreting them as danger or as proof that something is wrong in a relationship. Distress can feel intense and urgent, especially in the body.[2] Conversely, those with avoidant attachment often do the opposite—detaching from their inner cues or suppressing emotions.[3] This emotional distance can gradually make vulnerability, intimacy, and relying on others feel challenging.

### *Sense of Self*

Interoception plays a key role in developing our sense of self—the inner awareness of *This is me*. It provides direct access to the signals inside our body that influence how we feel at every moment. These sensations are deeply personal: your hunger, your flutter of nerves, your warmth toward someone you care about. When these cues are clear and understandable, we can connect them to what's happening around us, identify our own emotions, and distinguish them from others' feelings.[4] This blending of internal and external information helps form the stable sense of self that we carry into relationships.[5]

These abilities begin developing in infancy through the everyday rhythms of caregiving. Moment-to-moment exchanges—eye contact, vocal tone, touch, and soothing—help an infant learn their internal sensations belong to them: *my hunger*, *my discomfort*, *my calm*. When caregivers respond with consistency and emotional presence, children begin to recognize their own internal signals and tell them apart from what's happening around them.

When attachment is disrupted through inconsistency, emotional unavailability, or trauma, this early learning becomes blurred. Children may grow up unsure of what their bodily cues mean or feel overly influenced by others' emotions, because no one helped them make sense of those signals. With time, this can make it more difficult to develop a coherent, resilient sense of self.[6]

## Empathy and Interpersonal Connection

Empathy is the ability to understand and feel with another person—to see their perspective, connect with their emotions, and respond with care. Because our emotional life is closely tied to interoception, the two are inseparable. When we can recognize and interpret our own internal states, we're better able to meet others with presence, attunement, and authentic empathy. Interoception is one of the key pillars of safe and compassionate connection.

Research indicates that individuals who are more in tune with their internal sensations tend to show greater empathy—they can feel into another person's emotions while remaining grounded in themselves. Research suggests that when we try to understand what someone else is experiencing, our own body may subtly mirror aspects of their emotional state. This process, called *embodied cognition*, involves using our internal experience as a reference point for interpreting what others may be going through.[7] When interoceptive awareness is clear and regulated, it supports perspective-taking, emotional resonance, and compassionate connection. Essentially, the more connected we are to our bodies, the more receptive we become to genuine connection with others.

Being able to empathize with someone is only part of the story. We also need a clear sense of where we are within that experience—what we're feeling, what belongs to the other person, and how to stay connected without becoming overwhelmed or pulled too far away. Interoception helps us stay engaged with others while remaining grounded in ourselves. When this balance is disrupted, our interactions with others can shift in several ways.

### *Self–Other Distinction*

Interoception is essential in helping us recognize where we end and others begin. Feldman and colleagues describe internal sensations as gentle anchors—constant reminders that our bodies exist in space and have their own boundaries.[8] The support of the chair beneath you, the rhythm of your breath, or a flutter in your chest all signal *This is me*. When we lose connection with these internal cues, our sense of self can become less stable, and we may rely more on external signals—others' emotions, opinions, or expectations—to understand who we are.

This inner clarity is closely connected to empathy. People who are attuned to their bodily signals are often better at sensing what someone else is feeling without losing themselves in the process.[9] When we can differentiate our emotions from another's, we stay grounded enough to offer compassion instead of becoming overwhelmed. Empathy flourishes in that balance—feeling with someone while remaining rooted in our own experience. When that balance breaks down, we may absorb others' feelings and become overloaded or shut down to protect ourselves.

When internal awareness becomes harder to access, our sense of self and boundaries can become blurry. We might depend on others to tell us how we feel or who we are, struggle to express our needs, or find ourselves influenced by others' emotions more than our own.[10] In this way, interoception not only fosters connection—it helps us stay connected while remaining true to ourselves.

Trauma and insecure attachment, however, can interfere with this process. When interoceptive signals become confusing or dysregulated, accessing empathy becomes more difficult. Researchers note that trauma can create noisy internal cues, making it hard to tell whether a feeling is ours or someone else's.[11] This confusion can lead to overwhelm, numbing, or withdrawal—responses that protect in the moment but also make closeness feel risky.

People often assume that supporting others in healing from trauma is difficult. As a therapist, I have learned that the more I connect with my own internal experience, the easier it becomes to distinguish between my feelings and those of my clients. This awareness helps me stay present and compassionate without becoming overwhelmed. Instead of absorbing their emotions, I am able to be with them—with openness, steadiness, and genuine feeling. It has given me more capacity to share their joy, sorrow, or relief while remaining rooted in myself.

## *Enmeshment and Overidentification with Others*

It becomes easier to absorb others' emotions when the boundary between the self and other blurs. Although empathy helps us be present with another person, it can sometimes shift into overidentification with their feelings and experiences, leading us to take on emotions—such as sadness or anxiety—that belong to the other person. Poor emotional boundaries can also prompt people to suppress their own needs to keep the peace or to feel responsible for others being alright before they can relax. This pattern contributes to difficulty saying no and to caretaking behaviors. Children in unhealthy families may grow up feeling responsible for a parent's emotional needs or comfort, creating a role reversal that contributes to insecure attachment patterns.

> *Lauren often absorbs others' emotions as if they were her own. Her strong empathy helps her connect deeply, but it can tip into overidentification and caretaking. Being responsible for the well-being of her mother, who had MS, taught her that others' needs came first, creating a role reversal that shaped her anxious attachment. As an adult, she struggles to say no and tends to minimize her own needs to maintain harmony, often feeling accountable for others' emotions. As a result, she carries both her own stress and the emotional weight of others, making it harder to tune into her own signals and care for herself without guilt.*

## *Overextension and Narcissistic Behaviors*

When the distinction between self and others is weak, difficulties can emerge in very different ways. Instead of absorbing others' emotions or neglecting their own needs, some people may overidentify with themselves—unable to see where their feelings and desires end and someone else's begin. This can show up in narcissistic traits, where a person prioritizes their own view, ignores others' needs, or reacts strongly when boundaries are set. Rather than yielding to others' expectations, they tend to push past them.

Blurred boundaries between self and other can also affect how someone interprets social cues. Bouffard and Miller found that sexual arousal, for example, can distort perception, making people more likely to misinterpret interest or assume consent when there isn't any.[12] From an internal-awareness perspective, this suggests that when internal signals dominate, it becomes harder to distinguish between *what I'm feeling* and *what they are feeling*. In these moments, personal arousal may be mistaken for shared interest—illustrating how crucial clear internal boundaries are for respectful, attuned connection.

## A Nervous System Perspective on Relationships

Looking at relationships through a nervous system lens helps us see how deeply our bodies shape the way we connect. At any moment, subtle internal shifts—changes in breathing, heart rate, muscle tension, or gut sensations—interact with cues we pick up from others, such as their tone of voice, facial expressions, and physical presence. Together, these signals influence whether we feel open and at ease, alert and guarded, or overwhelmed and pulled away.

These shifts often happen before we consciously notice them. When our system feels calm and supported, connection comes more easily. When it feels stressed or overwhelmed, we move into protection. In this way, safety, closeness, empathy, and boundaries aren't just ideas; they're experiences we feel in our bodies.

### *How Early Patterns Shape Adult Relationships*

Clinician and neuroscientist Allan Schore describes attachment as fundamentally about learning to regulate emotion within a relationship. An infant cannot manage stress alone; through repeated experiences of being soothed and responded to, the child gradually learns what calm feels like. These early interactions shape how safety is sensed, how closeness feels, and how internal signals are interpreted in later relationships.[13]

When caregiving is consistent and responsive, the nervous system becomes more flexible. When it is unpredictable or traumatic, protective patterns—such as heightened reactivity or withdrawal—can become familiar coping strategies. These embodied patterns often continue to shape relationships and conflicts well into adulthood.

Much of our relational life still unfolds in the body. Before we have words, our bodies respond. A softened voice can ease tension; a harsh tone can tighten the chest; a warm glance can bring relief. These responses are automatic and deeply human. At the same time, we are sensing our own internal state. When interoception is steady and clear, we can distinguish between *I feel anxious* and *This situation is unsafe*. But when trauma, attachment wounds, chronic stress, or neurodiversity disrupt that clarity, the line can blur. The body may activate protective responses even when no real threat is present.

In relationships, this mismatch can lead to misunderstanding. Someone may pull away, become defensive, or shut down—not because they don't want connection, but because their nervous system is trying to keep them safe. A person experiencing interoceptive challenges might

- notice bodily tension and assume something is wrong in the relationship
- feel on alert in moments of closeness without knowing why
- experience connection as overwhelming rather than comforting
- miss warning cues and assume safety when caution would be wise

## *Misinterpreting Cues: When Protection Overrides Connection*

Relational misunderstandings often arise not from what others say or do, but from what our own nervous system thinks is happening. When internal dysregulation or chronic stress becomes someone's baseline, even neutral interactions can be filtered through a lens of threat.

A sigh may feel like rejection.

A pause may feel like judgment.

A text delay may feel like abandonment.

A loved one's request can feel like pressure.

A neutral expression might seem like anger.

When the autonomic nervous system registers danger *before* thought forms, the mind quickly creates a narrative to make sense of the state. In these moments, our bodily state is shaping the story of what we *believe* is happening.

As Antonio Damasio has described, the brain continually interprets signals from the body and assigns them meaning.[14] Interoceptive cues don't just inform us about what is happening physically—they influence how we feel and how we understand our experience. The state of the body helps shape the narrative of the mind.

When the body moves into heightened activation, the story may sound like:

*They're judging me.*

*I need to protect myself.*

*I can't trust this.*

When the body settles into shutdown—heavy, slowed, or disconnected—the story may shift toward:

*I don't matter.*

*There's no point.*

*I'm alone.*

But when the nervous system is more regulated and flexible, the narrative can soften:

*We can work through this.*

*I can stay present.*

*This feels manageable.*

When interoception is dysregulated, it becomes harder to notice the early bodily cues that something is shifting—so the emotional story arrives fully formed and feels absolute. We may not realize how our own internal state and the interoceptive cues driving it are shaping the story we tell ourselves.

*David's negative self-story is closely tied to his depressed, low-energy state. When his nervous system enters shutdown—heavy, numb, and disconnected—his thoughts take on the same tone. Fatigue and emotional blunting feed a story that he doesn't matter and there's no point in trying. He pulls away from his wife because he feels undeserving of closeness, and withdraws from his sons because he believes they're better off without him. His physiology isn't just affecting his mood—it's forming the story he tells about himself and his place in his family.*

Viewing relationship struggles through the body's perspective reveals that many interpersonal challenges are nervous system responses to perceived threat. When interoceptive cues signal danger, the body moves into a protective state before we even think. We may pull away, become defensive, shut down, or misread others' intentions. Recognizing how our internal states influence these reactions creates space for compassion—for ourselves and those we care about. As interoceptive awareness grows, we strengthen the mind–body connection, enabling us to respond from a place of safety rather than fear and opening the door to more ease and connection in our relationships.

## Loneliness

Nearly a quarter of people around the world report feeling lonely often.[15] Loneliness is now recognized as a significant public health concern, associated with a higher risk for both mental and physical health problems.[16] But loneliness is not only a thought or social circumstance—it is an embodied experience.

Lisa Quadt and colleagues describe interoception as a sensory bridge connecting the body and mind, one that can be disrupted in loneliness. The brain may start misreading internal cues about safety or connection, making someone feel more isolated than they actually are. This research also suggests that loneliness can function like a predictive processing error: The brain expects disconnection and begins interpreting internal discomfort as evidence of social rejection.[17] This can lead to withdrawal and reinforce painful emotional patterns over time.

The work of Quadt and her colleagues also highlights the body's role in sensing safety and connection. When loneliness takes hold, internal cues can become skewed toward danger. A nervous flutter in the chest may feel like a warning rather than excitement, and pulling away may seem safer than reaching out. If this pattern continues, the body's stress response stays activated, making emotions harder to regulate and social interactions more draining. Longing for connection and self-protection can coexist. In this way, loneliness isn't just an emotional experience—it is embodied. Prolonged disconnection can alter how the brain and body communicate, affecting health, mood, and our ability to connect with others.[18]

## How MAIA Domains Can Be Impacted in Interpersonal Difficulties

Although interpersonal challenges take many forms, they often stem from attachment disruptions, relational wounds, or a nervous system that struggles to stay regulated. When someone is caught in a chronic stress response or becomes more withdrawn and disconnected, relationships naturally become harder to navigate. The MAIA domains most impacted in these situations often include emotional awareness, self-regulation, and trust.

**Emotional Awareness.** This domain is frequently disrupted. When connection feels overwhelming or confusing, it becomes difficult to distinguish sensations from emotions or to understand what internal cues mean. Boundaries between self and others may blur, making it unclear whose feelings are whose. With limited emotional awareness, bodily signals can be misread, and the stories we tell ourselves about interactions may become distorted. Trouble linking sensations to emotions often sits at the heart of many relationship struggles.

**Self-Regulation.** Challenges with self-regulation often grow out of limited emotional awareness. Since interoceptive signals help us soothe and manage distress, disruptions here can affect our relationships. When early co-regulation was inconsistent, or when trauma pushed the nervous system into chronic fight-or-flight or shutdown, it becomes harder to notice early signs of dysregulation. In relationships, this means small cues can trigger outsized reactions, and calming down takes more effort. Without reliable interoceptive grounding, conflict escalates quickly, vulnerability feels risky, and even closeness can become overwhelming.

**Trust.** Trauma, inconsistent caregiving, loneliness, and attachment wounds can make people doubt the reliability of their internal signals. When the nervous system perceives danger, bodily cues may be misinterpreted as signs of relational threat, and patterns like shutdown, dissociation, or hypervigilance make it even harder to trust what the body is communicating. Many adults struggle to trust their instincts about closeness, vulnerability, or safety, leading them to pull away, guard themselves, or move back and forth between seeking connection and withdrawing. When the body feels untrustworthy, trusting others also becomes more difficult.

# Part Four

# WHAT WORKS

# 20

# Determining What's Helpful

We have covered what interoception is, why it matters in daily life, how it can become disrupted, and how those disruptions contribute to emotional and psychological distress. With that foundation in place, we can now begin to explore how interoceptive processes can be intentionally shaped and strengthened. No book on interoception would be complete without practical tools that support our capacity to listen to the ongoing mind–body conversation and better understand what our bodies are communicating.

Before we can discuss specific practices that build interoceptive awareness, it's important to clarify what these practices aim to change. To understand what works, we need a clear picture of the interoceptive skills that can be altered and how those alterations create distress. Throughout this book, the MAIA has offered a useful framework, emphasizing that interoception is not a single ability but a constellation of related skills. Improving interoceptive awareness starts with identifying which of these skills may benefit from more focused support.

While writing this book, I had the privilege of speaking with Dr. Wolf Mehling, the primary developer and researcher behind the MAIA, about incorporating the questionnaire. He emphasized the importance of communicating that low scores are not inherently pathological or maladaptive, noting that there are no established "normal" values. In other words, for anyone completing the questionnaire, it's meant to be an invitation to curiosity and self-reflection rather than a source of self-judgment.

## Multidimensional Assessment of Interoceptive Awareness (MAIA-2)

The MAIA-2 is the most recent version of a self-reflection questionnaire designed to explore how people notice, interpret, and relate to interoceptive cues.[1] It includes thirty-seven statements about bodily sensations, attention, and emotional awareness, organized across the eight MAIA domains. Completing it can offer a deeper understanding of your own experience of internal sensations. Your responses should reflect what is generally true for you, not what you think *should* be true—there are no right or wrong answers. If you prefer to take the online version of the assessment, you can do so at www.carriedejong.com/maia.

The MAIA-2 is not a medical or psychological test but a tool for understanding patterns of bodily awareness. It is scored by subscales rather than as a single total score, since each domain represents a distinct aspect of interoception. Some items are reverse-scored during calculation so that, after scoring, higher subscale scores consistently reflect greater interoceptive awareness.

## MULTIDIMENSIONAL ASSESSMENT OF INTEROCEPTIVE AWARENESS (MAIA-2)

### RESPONSE SCALE FOR ALL QUESTIONS:

0 = Never 1 = Rarely 2 = Sometimes 3 = Often 4 = Usually 5 = Always

### Noticing

#### AWARENESS OF UNCOMFORTABLE, COMFORTABLE, AND NEUTRAL BODY SENSATIONS

| | Never | | | | | Always |
|---|---|---|---|---|---|---|
| 1. When I am tense I notice where the tension is located in my body. | 0 | 1 | 2 | 3 | 4 | 5 |
| 2. I notice when I am uncomfortable in my body. | 0 | 1 | 2 | 3 | 4 | 5 |
| 3. I notice where in my body I am comfortable. | 0 | 1 | 2 | 3 | 4 | 5 |
| 4. I notice changes in my breathing, such as whether it slows down or speeds up. | 0 | 1 | 2 | 3 | 4 | 5 |

Scoring—Noticing

Add items 1–4 for a Total Score: ________

Divide the total by 4 for the **MAIA Noticing Score:** ________

## Not-Distracting

### TENDENCY NOT TO IGNORE OR DISTRACT ONESELF FROM SENSATIONS OF PAIN OR DISCOMFORT

| | Never | | | | | Always |
|---|---|---|---|---|---|---|
| 1. I ignore physical tension or discomfort until they become more severe. | 0 | 1 | 2 | 3 | 4 | 5 |
| 2. I distract myself from sensations of discomfort. | 0 | 1 | 2 | 3 | 4 | 5 |
| 3. When I feel pain or discomfort, I try to power through it. | 0 | 1 | 2 | 3 | 4 | 5 |
| 4. I try to ignore pain. | 0 | 1 | 2 | 3 | 4 | 5 |
| 5. I push feelings of discomfort away by focusing on something else. | 0 | 1 | 2 | 3 | 4 | 5 |
| 6. When I feel unpleasant body sensations, I occupy myself with something else so I don't have to feel them. | 0 | 1 | 2 | 3 | 4 | 5 |

**Scoring—Not-Distracting (Reverse scoring)**

Add items 1–6 for a Total Score: ________, then subtract that number from 30: ________

30 – Total Score = ________

Divide this number by 6 for the **MAIA Not-Distracting Score:** ________

## Not-Worrying

### TENDENCY NOT TO WORRY OR EXPERIENCE EMOTIONAL DISTRESS WITH SENSATIONS OF PAIN OR DISCOMFORT

| | Never | | | | | Always |
|---|---|---|---|---|---|---|
| 1. When I feel physical pain, I become upset. | 0 | 1 | 2 | 3 | 4 | 5 |
| 2. I start to worry that something is wrong if I feel any discomfort. | 0 | 1 | 2 | 3 | 4 | 5 |
| 3. I can notice an unpleasant body sensation without worrying about it. | 0 | 1 | 2 | 3 | 4 | 5 |
| 4. I can stay calm and not worry when I have feelings of discomfort or pain. | 0 | 1 | 2 | 3 | 4 | 5 |
| 5. When I am in discomfort or pain I can't get it out of my mind. | 0 | 1 | 2 | 3 | 4 | 5 |

**Scoring—Not-Worrying (Reverse scoring for questions 1, 2, and 5)**

Add items 1, 2, and 5 for Reverse Scoring: ________, then subtract that number from 15 = ________

Add items 3 and 4 for Nonreverse Scoring: ________

Reverse Scoring total + Nonreverse Scoring total = ________

Divide this number by 5 for the **MAIA Not-Worrying Score:** ________

## Attention Regulation

### ABILITY TO SUSTAIN AND CONTROL ATTENTION TO BODY SENSATIONS

| | Never | | | | | Always |
|---|---|---|---|---|---|---|
| 1. I can pay attention to my breath without being distracted by things happening around me. | 0 | 1 | 2 | 3 | 4 | 5 |
| 2. I can maintain awareness of my inner bodily sensations even when there is a lot going on around me. | 0 | 1 | 2 | 3 | 4 | 5 |
| 3. When I am in conversation with someone, I can pay attention to my posture. | 0 | 1 | 2 | 3 | 4 | 5 |
| 4. I can return awareness to my body if I am distracted. | 0 | 1 | 2 | 3 | 4 | 5 |
| 5. I can refocus my attention from thinking to sensing my body. | 0 | 1 | 2 | 3 | 4 | 5 |
| 6. I can maintain awareness of my whole body even when a part of me is in pain or discomfort. | 0 | 1 | 2 | 3 | 4 | 5 |
| 7. I am able to consciously focus on my body as a whole. | 0 | 1 | 2 | 3 | 4 | 5 |

**Scoring—Attention Regulation**

Add items 1–7 for a Total Score: ________

Divide the total by 7 for the **MAIA Attention Regulation Score:** ________

## Emotional Awareness

### AWARENESS OF THE CONNECTION BETWEEN BODY SENSATIONS AND EMOTIONAL STATES

| | Never | | | | | Always |
|---|---|---|---|---|---|---|
| 1. I notice how my body changes when I am angry. | 0 | 1 | 2 | 3 | 4 | 5 |
| 2. When something is wrong in my life I can feel it in my body. | 0 | 1 | 2 | 3 | 4 | 5 |
| 3. I notice that my body feels different after a peaceful experience. | 0 | 1 | 2 | 3 | 4 | 5 |
| 4. I notice that my breathing becomes free and easy when I feel comfortable. | 0 | 1 | 2 | 3 | 4 | 5 |
| 5. I notice how my body changes when I feel happy / joyful. | 0 | 1 | 2 | 3 | 4 | 5 |

### Scoring—Emotional Awareness

Add items 1–5 for a Total Score: ________

Divide the total by 5 for the **MAIA Emotional Awareness Score:** ________

## Self-Regulation

### ABILITY TO REGULATE DISTRESS BY ATTENTION TO BODY SENSATIONS

| | Never | | | | | Always |
|---|---|---|---|---|---|---|
| 1. When I feel overwhelmed I can find a calm place inside. | 0 | 1 | 2 | 3 | 4 | 5 |
| 2. When I bring awareness to my body I feel a sense of calm. | 0 | 1 | 2 | 3 | 4 | 5 |
| 3. I can use my breath to reduce tension. | 0 | 1 | 2 | 3 | 4 | 5 |
| 4. When I am caught up in thoughts, I can calm my mind by focusing on my body / breathing. | 0 | 1 | 2 | 3 | 4 | 5 |

### Scoring—Self-Regulation

Add items 1–4 for a Total Score: ________

Divide the total by 4 for the **MAIA Self-Regulation Score**: ________

### Body Listening

**ACTIVE LISTENING TO THE BODY FOR INSIGHT**

| | Never | | | | | Always |
|---|---|---|---|---|---|---|
| 1. I listen for information from my body about my emotional state. | 0 | 1 | 2 | 3 | 4 | 5 |
| 2. When I am upset, I take time to explore how my body feels. | 0 | 1 | 2 | 3 | 4 | 5 |
| 3. I listen to my body to inform me about what to do. | 0 | 1 | 2 | 3 | 4 | 5 |

Scoring—Body Listening

Add items 1–3 for a Total Score: ________

Divide the total by 3 for the **MAIA Body Listening Score:** ________

### Trusting

**EXPERIENCE OF ONE'S BODY AS SAFE AND TRUSTWORTHY**

| | Never | | | | | Always |
|---|---|---|---|---|---|---|
| 1. I am at home in my body. | 0 | 1 | 2 | 3 | 4 | 5 |
| 2. I feel my body is a safe place. | 0 | 1 | 2 | 3 | 4 | 5 |
| 3. I trust my body sensations. | 0 | 1 | 2 | 3 | 4 | 5 |

Scoring—Trusting

Add items 1–3 for a Total Score: ________

Divide the total by 3 for the **MAIA Trusting Score:** ________

## What Do Survey Scores Mean?

If you have completed the MAIA-2, you may experience a range of reactions: curiosity, recognition, surprise, or even uncertainty. All of these responses are understandable. As Dr. Mehling emphasized, there are no "normal" scores and no single pattern that defines a healthy or ideal way of sensing the body. Your scores simply reflect patterns shaped by learning, experience, and the environmental and cultural contexts you've been part of.

The interpretations that follow are meant to spark curiosity. They explain what each domain represents, highlight what may already be working well, and point to areas where there may be room for growth. Their purpose is to support reflection rather than self-judgment, emphasizing that interoceptive awareness is changeable and can evolve over time. These areas of potential growth may be especially helpful for anyone who recognizes that their interoceptive patterns could be contributing to the mental or physical health challenges discussed in earlier chapters.

**Noticing.** Interoceptive awareness begins with noticing bodily sensations such as breath, heartbeat, tension, or discomfort without immediately judging or interpreting them. This first scale reflects how readily you perceive physical sensations as they arise, whether they are pleasant, unpleasant, or neutral sensations.

Higher scores can mean

- a natural awareness of bodily signals
- an ability to detect subtle shifts, such as tension or changes in breathing
- a habit of checking in with your body throughout the day

Lower scores may reflect opportunities to

- bring more curiosity to everyday body sensations
- pause long enough to notice what your body is telling you
- increase awareness of sensations of ease, comfort, or neutrality

**Not-Distracting.** Another key aspect of interoceptive awareness is the ability to stay connected to bodily sensations—even uncomfortable ones—without avoiding them or distracting yourself. This domain assesses how you respond to physical discomfort: whether you remain present with it or quickly turn your attention elsewhere.

Higher scores can mean

- an easier time staying with bodily sensations, even when they are uncomfortable
- greater ability to tolerate discomfort without immediately turning away from it
- a willingness to listen before reacting

Lower scores may reflect opportunities to

- gently increase your tolerance for discomfort
- learn to stay with sensations for brief periods without needing to distract
- build trust that discomfort can be informative, not just something to escape

**Not-Worrying.** Interoceptive awareness also includes the ability to experience bodily sensations without worry or rumination. This domain reflects the extent to which emotional distress or worry accompanies physical sensations. It involves accepting sensations as they are and reducing the tendency to catastrophize about them.

Higher scores can mean

- a calmer relationship with bodily discomfort
- confidence that sensations can pass without needing to worry
- emotional flexibility when facing stressors

Lower scores may reflect opportunities to

- develop self-soothing skills
- learn to separate sensation from catastrophic interpretation
- strengthen the ability to describe a sensation without interpreting it

**Attention Regulation.** This domain reflects the ability to direct and keep attention on bodily sensations, even when distracted or busy. It involves choosing when and how to tune in, tracking sensations without becoming hypervigilant, and disengaging when attention becomes overwhelming.

Higher scores can mean

- increased flexibility in where your attention goes
- the ability to return awareness to the body when your mind wanders
- greater ease in shifting between thinking and sensing

Lower scores may reflect room to grow in

- practicing brief moments of body-focused attention
- strengthening the skill of turning attention inward and then outward
- gently redirecting attention back toward inner experience when your mind wanders

**Emotional Awareness.** Interoception involves noticing how bodily sensations connect to emotional experience. This domain reflects how well you recognize the physical cues of emotion in your body and how effectively you distinguish emotional sensations from other physical signals.

Higher scores can mean

- awareness of how emotions show up physically
- sensitivity to emotional shifts before they become overwhelming
- a stronger ability to differentiate among various emotions

Lower scores may reflect room to grow in

- exploring how emotions express themselves physically
- increasing your ability to describe the bodily sensations involved in emotional experiences
- learning to recognize emotional sensations more easily

**Self-Regulation.** This domain reflects how effectively you use body awareness to steady or soothe yourself during stress. Interoceptive cues can help you notice early signs of dysregulation and guide more supportive responses—such as resting, moving, eating, or setting boundaries. Rather than reacting automatically or suppressing sensations, the body becomes a source of information that can shape everyday self-care and decision-making.

Higher scores can mean

- access to internal calming resources
- the ability to settle the nervous system through breath or grounding tools
- confidence in using the body to help regulate

Lower scores may reflect room to grow in

- identifying and using body-based tools that help regulate the nervous system
- practicing calming strategies during low-stress moments
- learning to make small adjustments before stress escalates

**Body Listening.** This domain reflects how actively you listen to your body for information and guidance. Body listening involves paying attention to internal cues and sensations to better understand your needs and feelings, and allowing this information to direct your decisions, boundaries, and daily choices.

Higher scores can mean

- treating your body with greater compassion
- curiosity about the messages your body sends
- trust in bodily cues when making decisions

Lower scores may reflect room to grow in

- practicing how to listen for what your body is communicating
- slowing down enough to sense internal responses
- viewing bodily signals as useful sources of information

**Trusting.** This scale reflects your overall sense of safety, comfort, and trust in your body. It focuses on recognizing that most bodily sensations are not harmful, tend to rise and fall naturally, and can be tolerated without needing to control or avoid them. Over time, this trust supports a sense that the body has an innate ability to settle and regulate itself.

Higher scores can mean

- a sense of being "at home" in your body
- confidence in your bodily signals
- an embodied sense of safety

Lower scores may reflect room to grow in

- rebuilding safety and trust at your own pace
- developing gentle, positive bodily experiences
- allowing trust to emerge gradually

## Building Interoceptive Awareness with Care and Choice

Before we explore more specific ways to enhance interoceptive awareness, let's pause to reflect on some core principles about what *truly* builds interoceptive skills. These perspectives shape how these skills develop and clarify why some approaches are more effective than others. They can make the difference between merely trying techniques and genuinely cultivating a deeper, more adaptable ability to listen to the ongoing mind–body conversation.

As you explore different tools and start experimenting with them, the following principles can help guide your choices.

**Not all body-based practices develop interoceptive skills.**

Although many body-based practices—such as mindfulness, breathwork, yoga, and relaxation techniques—can be helpful, not all of them enhance interoceptive awareness equally. Some focus on noticing internal cues or responding to them in nonjudgmental ways. While these are valuable, they represent only part of interoceptive capacity.

Interoceptive awareness also includes how sensations are interpreted, how emotional responses are regulated, and whether the body is experienced as a reliable source of information. Some practices may increase sensation awareness without necessarily building comfort, confidence, or regulation.

The MAIA clarifies these distinctions by describing interoceptive awareness as a set of related but distinct skills. The value of scores across its eight domains is that they function like a roadmap for choosing or adapting practices that more precisely support the abilities someone wants to strengthen.

**Sustained attention can amplify distress rather than reduce it.**

For some individuals, especially those prone to anxiety or hypervigilance, sustained focus on bodily cues—such as heart rate or breath—can increase worry or reinforce anxiety-driven interpretations. In these cases, attention may become narrow and repetitive rather than curious and flexible. Instead of building interoceptive awareness, the practice may strengthen cycles of monitoring or fear of bodily sensations.

Interoceptive awareness benefits from having choices. Practices that encourage shifting attention among the body, the environment, and thoughts can be more helpful than those that require constant inward focus.

**More sensation awareness does not always mean more regulation.**

Some practices increase awareness of sensations without providing tools for emotional regulation or meaning-making. This can leave individuals feeling more vulnerable to internal signals and unsure how to respond. For instance, noticing tension without strategies for calming or interpretation may increase feelings of overwhelm rather than clarity. Awareness alone is often not enough; regulation tools and understanding are essential.

Interoceptive awareness is often easier to explore when combined with resources such as breath, movement, imagery, or external grounding. These supports can help create a felt sense of safety and choice.

**Meditation can sometimes lead to disconnection.**

Although meditation is often associated with a deeper connection to oneself, some individuals—especially those who have experienced trauma—may notice the opposite effect. Practices that emphasize stillness, inward attention, or prolonged observation can sometimes lead to dissociation, emotional numbness, or a feeling of checking out. These reactions are not signs that something is wrong; they often reflect protective patterns the nervous system has learned to rely on.

Some people experience stillness and silence as uncomfortable. You may find that movement, noticing your surroundings, or gentle sensory experiences offer an easier way to experiment with connection.

**Forcing attention inward can undermine trust in the body.**

Interoceptive awareness grows through invitation, not pressure. Practices that insist on "staying with" sensations despite distress may unintentionally strengthen the idea that the body must be controlled or endured. When people feel they need to push through discomfort to achieve awareness, trust in bodily signals may decrease rather than grow. Deepening interoceptive awareness is not measured by intensity or endurance.

The ability to trust bodily cues develops through opportunities for choice. When you can respect your need to notice a sensation, shift attention, or pause, the body is more likely to feel safe and reliable.

**For hypervigilant nervous systems, tracking discomfort can heighten distress rather than increase awareness.**

For individuals already highly attuned to bodily messages of discomfort, anxiety, or pain, interoceptive practices can unintentionally become exercises in vigilance rather than awareness. Attention may automatically shift toward sensations of discomfort—such as tightness in the chest, pain, or gastrointestinal sensations—and remain fixed there. When attention narrows around uncomfortable sensations, it can reinforce worry, fear-driven interpretations, or a sense that the body is unsafe. In these cases, the practice may increase distress rather than build understanding or regulation.

Interoceptive awareness is often more supportive when it doesn't focus solely on discomfort. For hypervigilant systems, skillful practice frequently involves expanding attention rather than narrowing it. If you notice attention becoming fixed on distressing sensations, it can be helpful to gently shift awareness to something neutral, steady, or mildly pleasant, such as

- the feeling of your feet making contact with the floor
- where your body meets the chair or surface beneath you
- the natural rhythm of the breath, without trying to change it

- a neutral area of the body that feels stable (e.g., the arms or feet)
- the sensations you notice when you gently rub your hands together

Shifting attention in this way isn't avoidance; it is a way of restoring balance. Moving attention toward neutral supports can help the nervous system settle, allowing interoceptive awareness to grow in a way that feels helpful rather than distressing. In time, this approach supports noticing discomfort without being pulled into it and directing attention in ways that foster regulation, trust, and safety.

**What works for one person may not work for everyone.**

Interoceptive ability is shaped by many factors, including stress, history, trauma, attachment styles, health, and environment. A practice that feels grounding and supportive for one person may feel activating or uncomfortable for another. One-size-fits-all approaches overlook individual differences in how nervous systems respond. Each nervous system is wired differently, and these differences are best met with curiosity and a willingness to listen. Approaching interoceptive practices with flexibility allows each person to discover what supports their own nervous system, at their own pace.

## Summing It Up and Moving Forward

It is helpful to remember that there is no quick, step-by-step guide to developing interoceptive skills. The MAIA framework and the principles outlined in this chapter offer a map rather than a single method. They clarify what interoceptive awareness involves, how individual differences shape experience, how skills can vary across domains, and why increasing bodily awareness doesn't necessarily improve well-being.

Understanding these distinctions matters. Without them, it's easy to assume that more attention is always better, meditation is always grounding, or discomfort must be endured for growth to occur. The MAIA reminds us that interoceptive awareness also depends on accurate interpretation, regulation, flexibility, and trust. With these principles in mind, we can now explore practices and tools that build greater capacity to listen to the vital communication unfolding within the body.

# 21

# Individual Practices

This chapter highlights specific practices that offer flexibility and emphasizes aspects of interoception that can be personalized. The tools presented are meant to be used selectively and adaptively, guided by the principles introduced in the previous chapter and by a growing understanding of your own interoceptive experience.

The first section provides several methods to intentionally practice the noticing of bodily sensations. The aim is to build skills related to curiosity, neutral observation, and awareness of internal bodily experiences. This section also includes two practices that show how a practice can be adapted to enhance awareness across the eight MAIA domains.

The rest of the chapter goes on to describe several additional categories of interoceptive-awareness practices, including those centered on breath, movement, and grounding.

## Body Tracking Practices

### *Quick Interoceptive Check-In*

A quick interoceptive check-in is a brief, ten-second pause to tune in to your body in the midst of everyday life. It is not a formal exercise—just a moment of noticing to build interoceptive awareness. You might sense your breath, posture, muscle tone, temperature, hunger, or a general feeling of ease or strain. It's about including your body in what you're already doing. A check-in can provide an opportunity to ask questions such as

- *What do I notice in my body right now?*
- *Am I energized, neutral, or calm?*

Because check-ins are short, they are less likely to feel overwhelming or onerous. They can also help reduce the tendency to analyze or overinterpret bodily cues. Check-ins can be done while waiting for someone, during a social interaction, sitting at your desk, or while out for a walk.

Depending on your intention and focus, this practice can support different MAIA domains. For example:

- ***What do I notice in my body right now?***
  Open, curious attention supports *Noticing.*
- ***Can I stay with this sensation for a few seconds without changing it?***
  Staying present with a body sensation supports *Not-Distracting.*
- ***Can I notice this sensation without judging or interpreting it?***
  Neutral observation reinforces *Not-Worrying.*
- ***Where do I feel my breath most clearly?***
  Steady, focused attention on the breath reflects *Attention Regulation.*
- ***Am I energized, neutral, or calm right now?***
  Checking in with overall emotional tone builds *Emotional Awareness.*
- ***If I track my breath for ten seconds, what happens inside?***
  Using breath intentionally can help with *Self-Regulation.*
- ***Is there a place in my body that is asking for attention?***
  Openness to what the body is communicating engages *Body Listening.*
- ***Can I listen for a few seconds and trust that it will be OK?***
  Confidence in pausing and listening reflects *Trusting.*

## Sensation Labeling

Sensation labeling is a quick exercise that enhances interoceptive awareness by using simple, neutral words to describe bodily sensations. It involves pausing for a few seconds to notice an internal sensation and name its quality, rather than interpreting its meaning.

This practice isn't about identifying emotions or explaining sensations; it's about naming them. Sensations may relate to breath, muscle tone, posture, temperature, internal processes, or a general sense of ease or tension. The goal is to describe what is present, just as it is, using everyday language. The next resource (The Language of Sensation) offers examples of words that can describe bodily sensations.

Sensation labeling can help reduce reactivity and overanalysis. Naming sensations often slows the nervous system and creates a small amount of space between the sensation and the urge to respond. This practice can be used during everyday activities.

Depending on your intention and how you engage in labeling, the same practice can also support different MAIA domains. For example:

- ***What word best describes what I feel right now?***
  Open, descriptive attention supports *Noticing*.
- ***Can I name this sensation and stay with it for a few seconds?***
  Staying present with a labeled sensation supports *Not-Distracting*.
- ***Can I describe this sensation without deciding what it means?***
  Using neutral language engages *Not-Worrying*.
- ***Can I track what happens after I label a sensation?***
  Sustaining attention reinforces *Attention Regulation*.
- ***What word describes the overall feeling in my body right now?***
  Labeling global sensations builds *Emotional Awareness*.
- ***If I name this sensation, does my body settle, activate, or remain neutral?***
  Noticing shifts supports *Self-Regulation*.
- ***Is there a sensation that stands out and wants to be named?***
  Responding to what draws attention engages *Body Listening*.
- ***Can I name what I feel and trust that my body knows how to handle it?***
  Labeling without urgency or control helps build *Trusting*.

* * *

## THE LANGUAGE OF SENSATION

This list includes words that describe how interoceptive sensations can feel inside the body, what's sometimes called the *felt sense*. These words offer simple ways to notice and name what is happening in the body in the present moment.

When we slow down and put words to bodily sensations, it can

- help us notice patterns in how the body responds to stress, safety, emotions, or thoughts
- increase body awareness without the need to analyze or fix anything
- make sensations feel more understandable and less overwhelming
- create language for experiences that are often hard to describe

There is no right or wrong word to describe your bodily sensations. You may notice more than one sensation at the same time, or you might notice very little.

You can use this list to

- gently scan the body and scc which words fit right now
- track how sensations shift over time
- distinguish among thoughts, emotions, and bodily sensations
- practice staying present with sensations rather than reacting to them

You may have additional words to add to this list. The goal is not precision—it is curiosity and connection with your body.

**Skin**

- Tingling
- Prickly
- Tight
- Crawling
- Sensitive
- Numb
- Raw
- Pulsing

**Breath**

- Shallow
- Deep
- Restricted
- Free
- Tight
- Smooth
- Expansive
- Labored

**Gastrointestinal**

- Queasy
- Fluttery
- Knotted
- Churning
- Heavy
- Full
- Tight
- Settled

**Whole Body**

- Heavy
- Light
- Collapsed
- Energized
- Disconnected
- Restless
- Still
- Frozen

**Emotional** *(These words describe how emotions can feel in the body, not the emotion itself.)*

- Tender
- Constricted
- Open
- Heavy
- Raw
- Tight
- Warm
- Expansive

**Intensity**

- Subtle
- Faint
- Strong
- Dull
- Sharp
- Surging
- Fading
- Steady

**Muscle**

- Tight
- Relaxed
- Trembling
- Weak
- Strong
- Sore
- Heavy
- Fatigued

**Temperature**

- Warm
- Cool
- Cold
- Chilled
- Flushed
- Burning
- Icy
- Radiating

**Heart / Chest**

- Pounding
- Fluttering
- Tight
- Open
- Heavy
- Calm
- Settled
- Warm

**Grounding / Orientation**

- Rooted
- Floating
- Anchored
- Wobbly
- Present
- Drifting
- Balanced
- Scattered

**Energy**

- Charged
- Drained
- Buzzing
- Flowing
- Blocked
- Dull
- Restless
- Calm

* * *

## *Localized Body Tracking*

Bring your attention to one area of the body (such as the chest, throat, or abdomen) and stay with it for about thirty to sixty seconds, allowing sensations to reveal themselves without trying to change anything. This is a quiet noticing practice—sensations such as temperature, movement, or stillness are all welcome.

- *What sensations are present here right now?* (Noticing)
- *Can I give this moment of sensation a little more time?* (Not-Distracting)
- *Does this sensation have an emotional tone?* (Emotional Awareness)
- *What happens if I stay a little longer?* (Self-Regulation)
- *If this sensation had a message, what might it be?* (Body Listening)
- *What feels supportive about noticing this?* (Trusting)

## *Body Scan*

Slowly move your attention through different regions of the body, noticing sensations as they arise. The purpose is to bring awareness to bodily experiences as you explore different areas. The goal is not to relax or change anything but to cultivate awareness, kindness, and a nonjudgmental attitude toward whatever is present.

- *Where do I notice sensations most clearly?* (Noticing)
- *What happens if I don't rush past this?* (Not-Distracting)
- *Is it possible to meet this with neutrality or kindness?* (Not-Worrying)

- *What helps me move my focus slowly and steadily?* (Attention Regulation)
- *Does my body need anything in this moment?* (Body Listening)
- *What feels supportive as I move through the body?* (Trusting)

### Noticing Comfortable and Neutral Body Sensations

Gently direct your attention to comfortable or neutral sensations in your body, without comparing them to anything else. This can be especially helpful if you tend to focus on discomfort or tension. Paying attention to neutral or supportive sensations can help balance awareness and reduce stress. If this feels difficult, try focusing on your hands or feet, or on the support of the chair beneath you. The goal isn't to avoid discomfort, but to strengthen your ability to notice comfort and neutrality as well.

- *Where do I notice ease or neutrality most clearly?* (Noticing)
- *Can I stay with this sensation for a few moments?* (Not-Distracting)
- *Is it OK if I focus on comfort for a few moments?* (Not-Worrying)
- *What helps me stay connected here?* (Attention Regulation)
- *How does my emotional state shift as I notice this?* (Emotional Awareness)
- *What feels supportive as I notice comfortable or neutral sensations?* (Trusting)

## Breath Tracking Practices

### Natural Breath Observation

Take a moment to notice where you feel your breath, without trying to regulate or change it. Your attention may be drawn to the rise and fall of your abdomen or chest, or to the sensation of air moving through your nostrils. The goal is simply to experience the breath as a bodily process and observe what it feels like to breathe.

- *Where do I feel the breath most clearly right now?* (Noticing)
- *Can I let the breath be natural, even if it feels uneven?* (Not-Worrying)
- *When my attention wanders, can I gently return to the breath?* (Attention Regulation)
- *How does my emotional state show up in the breath?* (Emotional Awareness)
- *Is there one area of my body where it feels easier to track my breath?* (Body Listening)
- *Can I trust my breath to take care of itself?* (Trusting)

### Longer Exhale Breath

Allow your exhale to be slightly longer than your inhale, in a gentle, natural way. You might breathe in for a few counts and out for a few more, keeping the breath smooth and relaxed. A longer exhale can help the body settle and feel calmer. There's no need to force or control the breath—adjust as needed so it remains comfortable.

- *What do I notice as the exhale lengthens slightly?* (Noticing)
- *Can I stay with the sensation of the exhale until it completes?* (Not-Distracting)
- *Is it OK to adjust if this feels like too much?* (Not-Worrying)
- *Does this way of breathing affect my overall state?* (Self-Regulation)
- *What length of exhale feels supportive rather than forced?* (Body Listening)
- *Can I trust my body to tell me when it's time to stop?* (Trusting)

### Hand-to-Heart / Hand-to-Belly Breathing

Place a hand on your chest or belly and allow the breath to move naturally beneath it. You may notice warmth, pressure, movement, or other sensations through the contact. This practice uses gentle touch to support awareness and regulation, without needing to change the breath in any way.

- *Is it OK if my breath feels uneven or subtle?* (Not-Worrying)
- *What happens if I let my hand rest here?* (Not-Distracting)
- *Can I gently return my attention to the sensation beneath my hand?* (Attention Regulation)
- *Does this touch bring up any feeling?* (Emotional Awareness)
- *Does placing my hand here affect how settled I feel?* (Self-Regulation)
- *Does my body prefer the hand on the chest or the belly?* (Body Listening)

## Movement-Based Practices

### Stretch–Release Cycles

Experiment with alternating between a mild stretch of your choosing and an easy release, moving only within a comfortable range. As the body stretches and then softens, see if you can track the sensations of effort and letting go.

The intention is to notice how the body experiences activation and release through movement.

- *What do I notice as I release?* (Noticing)
- *Can I stay with the sensations of effort and release?* (Not-Distracting)
- *Can I let this movement be comfortable rather than perfect?* (Not-Worrying)
- *Can I track the moment of transition from stretch to release?* (Attention Regulation)
- *Does this movement help my body feel more settled?* (Self-Regulation)
- *How much stretch feels supportive rather than straining?* (Body Listening)

## Weight-Shifting Awareness

Slowly shift your weight from one foot to the other, moving slowly enough to notice changes in pressure and balance. You may observe sensations in the feet, legs, hips, or spine as the weight transfers. The goal isn't to correct posture, but to sense how the body organizes itself through movement and support.

- *Where do I feel pressure or support most clearly?* (Noticing)
- *What happens if I slow this down?* (Not-Distracting)
- *Is it OK if this feels uneven or subtle?* (Not-Worrying)
- *Does this movement bring up a particular emotional tone?* (Emotional Awareness)
- *Does feeling my weight on the ground help me feel more settled?* (Self-Regulation)
- *Can I trust my body to find balance?* (Trusting)

## Interoceptive Walking

Walk at a relaxed pace while paying attention to internal sensations of movement. Your awareness may rest on foot pressure, muscle activity in the legs or arms, shifts in weight, or subtle internal changes with each step. The goal is not to alter how you walk, but to sense walking by paying attention to how it feels.

- *Where do I notice the movement most clearly?* (Noticing)
- *Can I stay with the sensations of walking rather than the goal?* (Not-Distracting)

- *What feeling emerges as I move?* (Emotional Awareness)
- *What shifts as I continue walking with awareness?* (Self-Regulation)
- *Does my body want to slow down or speed up?* (Body Listening)
- *Can I trust my body to move efficiently on its own?* (Trusting)

## Grounding Tools

### Hand Over Area of Activation

Gently place your hand over an area of discomfort, such as your chest or belly, and let it rest without pressure. Notice the sensations beneath your hand—warmth, contact, or movement. The goal is to stay present with the sensation while offering steadiness, without trying to change it.

- *What do I feel beneath my hand right now?* (Noticing)
- *Is it OK to let this sensation be present?* (Not-Worrying)
- *What happens if I keep my attention here?* (Not-Distracting)
- *What feeling, if any, is present as I rest my hand here?* (Emotional Awareness)
- *Does my body prefer a different placement?* (Body Listening)
- *Can I trust this simple contact to offer support?* (Trusting)

### Butterfly Tapping

Sit comfortably and take a breath or two to settle. Cross your arms over your chest, placing your hands palms down, with fingertips resting just below the opposite collarbones, like butterfly wings. Slowly tap, alternating left and right. Notice the sensations created by the rhythm and movement. Continue as long as it feels calming and grounding.

- *Can I stay with the sensations created by this rhythm?* (Not-Distracting)
- *Can I track the alternating pattern from side to side?* (Attention Regulation)
- *Does this tapping influence how I feel emotionally?* (Emotional Awareness)
- *What changes in my level of activation?* (Self-Regulation)
- *What pressure feels most supportive right now?* (Body Listening)
- *What feels steady as I practice this tapping?* (Trusting)

## Grounded Sitting

Sit comfortably and bring attention to the sensations you notice where your body makes contact with the chair. Notice how your weight is supported through the seat, legs, and along the spine. The intention is not to hold any particular posture, but to sense how the body is held and supported in this moment. Try relaxing slightly and letting the chair support you a bit more.

- *Where do I notice sensations of sitting most clearly?* (Noticing)
- *Can I stay with these contact sensations for a few moments?* (Not-Distracting)
- *Can I let my body relax slightly without the need to brace?* (Not-Worrying)
- *Does relaxing slightly change how my body feels?* (Self-Regulation)
- *Where could I soften or let go just a little?* (Body Listening)
- *Can I trust the chair to support me if I relax?* (Trusting)

# 22

# Practitioner-Led Therapies and Approaches

In the previous two chapters, you've had the opportunity to explore your own patterns of interoceptive awareness and experiment with practices that enhance your mind–body connection. You've also been encouraged to notice what feels helpful for you and your nervous system. As you've probably discovered, there is no single "right" way to develop interoceptive awareness.

You may now be interested in exploring other support or therapeutic options. The same principle applies—there's no one-size-fits-all solution. While no single method can guarantee resolving disconnection patterns or healing trauma entirely, many therapeutic approaches thoughtfully incorporate interoceptive awareness and provide meaningful ways to strengthen the mind–body connection. This chapter offers an overview of several practitioner-led approaches, including interoceptive work, to help you begin exploring what might resonate with you.

This information is intended as a guide. Listing these therapies does not mean I endorse one approach over another, nor does it suggest that any specific option will work for everyone. Think of this section as a starting point—a map you can use as you learn, research, and reflect on what might support your well-being. If something sparks your interest or curiosity, you might choose to explore further, speak with a trained practitioner, or try related practices at your own pace. The "best" approach is ultimately the one that feels safe, accessible, and aligned with your needs, readiness, and circumstances.

## Mindfulness and Interoception: Connected but Different

Interoceptive resources almost always include mindfulness practices. At first glance, this makes sense. Mindfulness has become increasingly popular in both research and daily life, and the term now encompasses a wide range of approaches that involve intentionally paying attention to the present moment. Many mindfulness practices emphasize noticing thoughts, bodily sensations, or the environment without rushing to judge them. In essence, mindfulness combines simple awareness with curiosity and acceptance. It can take the form of formal practices—such as body-awareness exercises or self-compassion meditations—or everyday activities, like paying attention while washing dishes or eating.

For these reasons, mindfulness offers a flexible set of attentional skills that can support interoceptive work. However, its usefulness depends on how those skills are introduced and used. Also, while mindfulness and interoceptive awareness share certain skills, they serve distinct purposes.

Mindfulness and interoceptive awareness often overlap, but they are not the same. It can be helpful to think of mindfulness as a way of paying attention. Interoceptive awareness, by contrast, involves a set of skills that allow a person to sense, interpret, tolerate, and use internal bodily sensations for emotional and behavioral regulation. Recognizing this distinction is crucial when considering which practices will truly enhance interoceptive capacity. Not all mindfulness practices focus on the body; many center on observing thoughts, feelings, or external stimuli. While these approaches can be beneficial, they are not designed to strengthen the specific interoceptive abilities measured by the MAIA.

Research by Hanley and colleagues helps clarify this distinction. Using both mindfulness measures and the MAIA, they found that mindfulness and interoceptive awareness are related but form separate clusters of skills.[1] Mindfulness influences how someone pays attention, encouraging qualities like nonjudgment and curiosity. The MAIA domains, in contrast, capture what a person notices in their body, how they interpret sensations, and whether they can use bodily information to guide regulation. Both are valuable, but each contributes something unique to well-being: Mindfulness shapes the quality of attention, while interoceptive awareness shapes the meaning and use of bodily signals.

While mindfulness can be a powerful tool for improving how people relate to bodily sensations, it is not a complete interoceptive training program on its own. Mindfulness practices that involve sustained attention to bodily experience can support interoceptive development, but mindfulness alone does not consistently cultivate the full range of interoceptive skills described in the MAIA.

## Mindfulness Is Not Always Safe or Effective for Trauma Survivors

Jonathan Gibson's trauma-focused research offers an important caution. For people with trauma histories—especially those who learned early in life to disconnect from bodily sensations—mindfulness practices that focus inward can sometimes trigger dissociation rather than awareness.[2] What may appear to be acceptance or calm can instead reflect emotional numbing or shutdown. In such cases, mindfulness does not improve interoceptive awareness; it may reinforce protective habits that block access to bodily signals and increase anxiety about engaging with physical sensations.

Depending on the individual, their nervous system, and the unique ways trauma responses are held in the body, body-focused interventions can feel overwhelming or destabilizing. Some individuals may not yet be able to tolerate sustained internal attention. For these people, slow, gradual exposure to bodily sensations within a supportive therapeutic relationship is not just helpful, it is essential. A therapist can monitor signs of dissociation, safely introduce body-based work, and support the gradual development of trust in inner experience. Without this support, mindfulness may feel confusing, unsafe, or even retraumatizing.

## Structured Mindfulness Programs

When exploring mindfulness practices that build interoceptive skills, it's helpful to remember that no single approach works for everyone. Research shows that mindfulness can improve certain aspects of interoception, but this typically occurs when practices are intentionally introduced and tailored to a person's nervous system, history, and needs. The goal is not to force a particular technique, but to identify what genuinely strengthens interoceptive awareness in ways that feel safe, regulating, and beneficial.

Although mindfulness alone is not a complete interoceptive training method, structured mindfulness-based programs offer more systematic approaches for developing mindful attention and emotion regulation. Programs like Mindfulness-Based Stress Reduction (MBSR), mindfulness-based cognitive therapy (MBCT), and acceptance and commitment therapy (ACT) offer clear structures, guided practices, and therapeutic support. Their organized format helps individuals apply mindful awareness more consistently. While each program emphasizes different elements, all aim to help people notice and relate to their internal experiences with greater clarity and stability—laying a strong foundation that can support and improve interoceptive skills.

**Mindfulness-Based Stress Reduction (MBSR).** This eight-week, nonreligious group program was developed by Jon Kabat-Zinn in the late 1970s to help people relate to stress more effectively. Through practices such as meditation, body scans, gentle stretching, and integrating mindfulness into daily life, participants learn to become more aware of their thoughts, emotions, and bodily sensations. This growing awareness supports key skills like present-moment attention, emotional regulation, nonreactivity, and compassion for oneself and others.

Research shows that MBSR can reduce anxiety, depression, and burnout; improve attention, emotional balance, resilience, and interpersonal functioning; and enhance performance in work and relationships. Physically, MBSR has been associated with better sleep, lower blood pressure and cortisol levels, stronger immune function, and reduced chronic pain. It has been used to support treatment of various health and mental health concerns, including chronic pain, substance use disorders, eating disorders, and mood and anxiety disorders.[3]

MBSR can help improve interoceptive awareness in several ways:

- It encourages individuals to direct attention to bodily sensations in a nonjudgmental, present-moment way.
- Practices such as body scans and mindful breathing help strengthen the ability to notice and sustain attention on specific sensations.
- People are encouraged to meet bodily sensations—even uncomfortable ones—with openness and curiosity rather than avoidance or worry, helping build a more accurate sense of the body's internal state.
- Enhanced self-awareness helps interrupt automatic responses to stress, emotions, or bodily cues and increases the ability to make conscious choices about how to respond to internal signals, including tension, discomfort, and emotion-based sensations.
- A strengthened ability to link body sensations with emotional states helps people identify emotions earlier and more accurately, enabling more adaptive use of emotion regulation strategies.

**Mindfulness-Based Cognitive Therapy (MBCT).** MBCT is derived from MBSR. It blends mindfulness practices with cognitive therapy tools to help people change how they relate to their thoughts and emotions. Instead of trying to push away or fight negative thoughts, MBCT teaches people to notice them with curiosity and without judgment. The program includes practices such as breathing meditation, body scans, gentle awareness of physical sensations, observing thoughts as mental events rather than facts, and exercises that build emotional balance. These skills help people recognize early signs of stress or low mood and respond in healthier, more skillful ways. MBCT has been shown to reduce symptoms of depression, anxiety, and stress and to support improved emotional regulation. Studies also show benefits for conditions such as bipolar disorder, PTSD, chronic pain, and cardiovascular disease.[4]

MBCT can lead to improvements in interoceptive awareness similar to those seen with MBSR, with additional skills that include

- nonjudgmental observation—noticing thoughts, feelings, and bodily sensations without reacting to or judging them, allowing sensations to be observed without avoidance or distraction
- breaking patterns of rumination—shifting attention to the "here and now" helps decrease dysfunctional cycles of negative, self-related thinking

**Acceptance and Commitment Therapy (ACT).** ACT focuses on six key skills that help build increased psychological flexibility. It supports individuals in staying present, open, and engaged in meaningful action. ACT teaches experiential acceptance and curiosity, which involves actively allowing thoughts, emotions, and bodily sensations without trying to avoid or change them. Cognitive defusion is a skill that helps people step back from their thoughts—seeing them as passing experiences rather than literal truths—through exercises that shift how one relates to thinking rather than trying to challenge or replace thoughts. ACT also encourages mindful awareness of the present moment, helping individuals notice what's happening right now with greater clarity. It includes self-as-context, a way of accessing a stable observer perspective so that difficult inner experiences can be noticed safely rather than becoming overwhelming.[5]

Although ACT does not explicitly target interoceptive awareness, its core skills help develop capacities that contribute to healthy interoception:

- **Acceptance** increases the willingness to notice bodily sensations long enough to observe and understand them accurately.

- **Mindfulness exercises** encourage individuals to notice what is happening in their bodies in the present moment, without judgment or avoidance.
- **Cognitive defusion** decreases the tendency to catastrophize thoughts, emotions, and bodily cues, which can intensify both anxious thoughts and distressing sensations.
- **Interoceptive exposure** involves being willing to allow and notice uncomfortable sensations, which builds tolerance and familiarity with unpleasant interoceptive cues.

## Somatic Psychotherapies and Body-Based Approaches

Somatic psychotherapy is a form of body-centered therapy—*soma* is the Greek word for *body*. Approaches in this category include the body in the healing process, recognizing that emotions, trauma, and stress are held in the physical body and nervous system. In addition to addressing trauma, somatic methods are effective for anxiety, stress, dissociation, emotional numbing, and interoceptive disruptions.

Somatic methods use techniques involving body awareness, movement, breath, and sensory experiences to help individuals process emotions, regulate the nervous system, and resolve emotional distress. Core features of somatic approaches include

- body awareness—noticing sensations, breath, tension, and movement
- enhanced mind–body integration—understanding how thoughts, emotions, and body sensations influence each other
- trauma healing—assisting the nervous system in recovering from trauma
- experiential techniques—methods that use body-based practices, movement, or hands-on approaches

Clinicians trained in somatic healing methods often draw on a variety of tools and techniques, combining multiple approaches. For example, a trained EMDR (eye movement desensitization and reprocessing) clinician might incorporate mindfulness-based interventions alongside other body-based therapies.

**Somatic Experiencing (SE).** SE is a gentle, body-based approach to healing trauma developed by Peter Levine. It is grounded in the idea that when a traumatic event interrupts the body's natural fight-or-flight response, the residual activation can become stuck in the nervous system. SE helps individuals notice their bodily sensations slowly and safely so the body can release held energy and complete protective responses that were never given the chance to unfold.[6]

SE uses interoceptive awareness as a central pathway for healing. By noticing subtle sensations such as breath, tightness, warmth, or tingling, people learn what activation and settling feel like in their own bodies. This strengthens the nervous system's capacity to self-regulate and lays a foundation for resilience.

The process unfolds gradually through a bottom-up approach. Instead of diving into the full trauma narrative, SE works with small, manageable shifts in sensation. Therapists guide clients in gently moving between activation and calm—a rhythm called *pendulation*. This pacing reduces overwhelm, prevents dissociation, and allows the body to discharge tension and return to balance naturally.

SE supports interoceptive awareness by

- introducing interoceptive cues gradually, without overwhelming the system
- using gentle pacing to make bodily sensations feel safer and clearer
- helping individuals reconnect with internal cues and rebuild a sense of safety and control, fostering emotional and physical resilience

**Eye Movement Desensitization and Reprocessing (EMDR)**. EMDR is a structured, trauma-focused therapy that helps people heal by reprocessing distressing memories. During EMDR, the individual briefly focuses on a traumatic memory while also engaging in bilateral stimulation—typically eye movements, taps, or sounds. This dual attention helps the brain lessen the intensity and emotional charge of the memory, reduce symptoms like flashbacks or nightmares, and integrate more adaptive beliefs about the event.

The treatment process follows an eight-phase protocol that incorporates various aspects of interoceptive awareness into the therapeutic plan, treating the body as a crucial part of how traumatic memories are stored and healed. During therapy, individuals are guided to notice shifts in sensations such as tension, tightness, or numbness. EMDR helps them gently reconnect with these sensations in a safe, structured manner. Over time, this supports a clearer understanding of bodily cues, reduces fear of internal sensations, and fosters a more grounded and regulated relationship with the body.

Many aspects of EMDR promote interoceptive awareness:

- Body scans are used to identify tension or distress.
- Exploring the felt sense of traumatic memories helps individuals attend to physical, emotional, and cognitive components.
- Observing changes in internal sensations strengthens awareness of shifting bodily cues.
- Controlled, gradual noticing of sensations reduces overwhelm, especially for individuals who experience dissociation.
- Building body-based resources, including interoceptive "anchors of safety" such as warmth or grounding sensations, supports regulation.
- Interoceptive exposure helps make feared or confusing body sensations feel less threatening.

**Sensorimotor Psychotherapy (SP).** SP is a therapeutic approach developed by Pat Ogden that recognizes the body as a vital source of information about a person's history and emotional life. Many therapists integrate SP with other modalities to ensure the body is included in the healing process. SP follows a three-phase model: (1) safety and stabilization, (2) processing, and (3) integration. It relies on close collaboration between therapist and client. Throughout the work, the therapist attends closely to the client's nervous system and bodily signals to keep the process safe and prevent overwhelm.[7]

People dealing with anxiety, trauma symptoms, attachment wounds, or persistent negative self-beliefs often feel stuck or discouraged. SP helps by focusing on the body's natural movements, posture, and internal sensations as pathways to understanding and shifting long-standing patterns. By slowing down and noticing cues such as tension, breath changes, or impulses to move, clients begin to uncover automatic physical and emotional habits that operate outside awareness. Through gentle experimentation and mindful tracking, SP supports the reorganization of these patterns and the development of new capacities for safety, connection, and resilience.

A core part of SP is strengthening interoceptive awareness by

- noticing defensive responses such as bracing or shutting down and recognizing internal signals of fear or activation

- exploring how posture and movement connect to past experiences and beliefs
- engaging in practices such as somatic tracking, breath awareness, and movement experiments to deepen interoceptive awareness and support healing

**A Nervous System–Informed Perspective.** This approach involves understanding how the body responds to stress and safety. It isn't a separate method but a viewpoint that can be integrated into approaches such as EMDR, somatic therapies, and other trauma-informed practices. The basic truth is simple: Healing becomes easier when the body feels safe and more regulated.

Trauma and chronic stress can leave the nervous system on high alert or prone to shutting down. These responses are not signs of weakness; they are protective patterns shaped by experience. Therapy helps clients recognize these patterns, understand their triggers, and gradually build skills to find more regulated states.

Together, therapist and client begin to "map" the nervous system—identifying stress triggers, noticing bodily cues of tension or withdrawal, and recognizing moments of calm or connection. This shared understanding makes reactions feel less confusing and more manageable. Over time, clients practice tools such as grounding, breath awareness, movement, and mindful tracking. The goal is not to eliminate stress responses but to expand flexibility and increase the capacity to move through different states with greater awareness and choice.

This lens also helps strengthen and support interoception by helping clients

- notice internal cues like breath, heart rate, and muscle tension
- develop language for different bodily states
- track sensations with curiosity rather than fear
- understand reactions as protective rather than personal flaws
- recognize cues of calm and connection, not just stress

**Trauma-Sensitive or Trauma-Informed Yoga (TIY).** TIY is a therapeutic adaptation of traditional yoga that emphasizes physical and psychological safety for people with trauma histories. Rather than prioritizing fitness, flexibility, spiritual practices, or relaxation, TIY centers on self-regulation, agency, and the restoration of the mind–body connection.[8] It avoids practices like hands-on adjustments, directive commands, or pressure to perform movements, instead using invitational, choice-based language so participants can engage at their own pace.

A central goal of TIY is to restore the capacity to notice and interpret internal bodily sensations, an ability often disrupted by trauma. Through gentle postures, breath awareness, and mindful attention to sensation, TIY helps increase tolerance for physiological states, reconnect individuals with their bodies, and enhance emotional regulation. Overall, TIY emphasizes the body—rather than verbal processing—as the primary pathway for healing, creating a safe and empowering space where people who have experienced trauma can regain a sense of autonomy, agency, and embodied self-connection.[9]

Research shows that TIY supports interoceptive awareness in several ways, including

- creating a safe, choice-based environment that encourages noticing bodily cues
- utilizing gentle guidance to help participants observe sensations, breath, and internal shifts without pressure
- engaging in repetitive sensation-focused practice to enhance body awareness and self-regulation
- supporting reconnection with the body, fostering a clearer and more coherent sense of self
- strengthening the ability to discern internal cues, make decisions based on sensations, and regulate emotions[10]

## Dialectical Behavior Therapy

Dialectical behavior therapy (DBT) is an evidence-based treatment developed from cognitive behavioral therapy (CBT) to help individuals regulate emotions, reduce harmful behaviors, and navigate life more effectively. The term *dialectical* reflects DBT's emphasis on balancing two ideas: accepting one's thoughts and feelings while also committing to meaningful change.[11]

A core goal of DBT is increasing awareness of internal experiences so individuals can respond rather than react to distress. Skills training is delivered in structured classes focused on mindfulness, distress tolerance, emotion regulation, and maintaining boundaries and self-respect in relationships. Emotion regulation in DBT depends on noticing both emotional cues and physical cues such as stress, fatigue, and pain. With practice, clients become more aware of bodily markers like muscle tension, changes in heart rate, and shifts in breathing, allowing earlier intervention before emotions escalate or harmful behaviors occur.

DBT is especially helpful in conditions where interoception is altered, including anxiety, depression, self-harm, PTSD, disordered eating, and substance misuse. For example:

- Clients learn to recognize rising emotional and physical arousal that can lead to urges for self-harm or substance use.
- Mindfulness and grounding help traumatized individuals reduce dissociation and reconnect with their bodily signals.
- Clients with eating disorders practice identifying hunger and fullness and distinguishing between physical and emotional cues.

## Occupational Therapy

Occupational therapists (OTs) help people of all ages who experience physical, emotional, cognitive, or developmental challenges that make daily activities more difficult. Their work focuses on supporting individuals in meaningful tasks—such as self-care, work, school activities, and social interactions—by enhancing key skills, modifying environments, and teaching practical strategies. OTs work with a diverse range of clients, from adults recovering from stroke or injury to those dealing with anxiety, depression, or trauma. They also support children with developmental delays, autism, sensory processing differences, or learning challenges, helping them build the motor, play, school, and self-care skills necessary for everyday participation.

A central part of occupational therapy involves addressing interoceptive challenges. OTs have long incorporated interoceptive tools into their practice because interoception is foundational for managing daily routines, self-care, learning, social engagement, and overall health. Interoceptive awareness helps individuals respond appropriately to cues such as hunger, stress, fatigue, pain, and toileting needs. To assess these skills, OTs use measures like the MAIA-2 for adults and structured, play-based interoception programs for children.

For adults, interoception-focused methods can enhance emotional regulation, stress management, and everyday functioning, particularly for those with trauma histories, mental health concerns, or difficulties with daily tasks. Strategies may include body-based sensory activities, mindfulness-based practices, and routines that strengthen the connection between bodily states, emotions, and actions. For children, therapists use structured programs, playful activities, and trauma-informed approaches to help them become more aware of their bodily sensations, link those sensations with emotions, and develop self-regulation skills. Across the lifespan, interoception-focused occupational therapy helps people better understand their bodies, feel more grounded, and participate more fully in meaningful daily activities.

## Interoceptive Exposure

Interoceptive exposure (IE) is a cognitive-behavioral technique that intentionally triggers physical sensations commonly associated with anxiety, panic, PTSD, and certain health conditions like chronic pain or IBS. Through specific exercises, individuals deliberately evoke bodily discomfort to help reduce distress and fear over time. Although inducing discomfort may seem counterintuitive, this method is strongly supported by research, particularly for panic disorder, as noted by Samantha Farris and colleagues.[12]

Their work shows that panic disorder is one of the most well-established applications of interoceptive exposure. In this condition, individuals develop a learned fear of bodily sensations after repeated distressing experiences, so even mild physical changes—such as a racing heart or shortness of breath—can trigger intense anxiety. This cycle of panic is maintained by catastrophic interpretations of these sensations. Interoceptive exposure directly interrupts this pattern by using structured, safe exercises that intentionally elicit feared sensations and allow individuals to experience them without avoidance. Over time, people realize that the feared outcomes do not happen and that they can tolerate and manage physical discomfort.[13]

Although the strongest evidence for the effectiveness of IE comes from studies on panic disorder and other anxiety disorders, research also supports its usefulness for symptoms of PTSD, health anxiety, and irritable bowel syndrome. Because fear and avoidance of bodily sensations contribute to many mental and physical health issues, the authors argue that interoceptive exposure is broadly relevant whenever distress results from misinterpreting or avoiding internal sensations.[14]

Farris and colleagues also found that interoceptive exposure is safe and well-tolerated. Temporary discomfort during exercises was common but expected and comparable to other exposure-based treatments, addressing concerns that intentionally inducing bodily sensations is harmful.[15]

* * *

You now have a variety of therapeutic options to explore if you're seeking additional support. You might continue with practices that have already been helpful, try a modality described in this chapter, or connect with a practitioner whose approach matches your needs. There are many ways to listen to your body and strengthen the interoceptive dialogue that promotes emotional and mental health. May the information in these chapters encourage you to pursue what feels supportive as you continue developing a compassionate relationship with your own body.

# 23

# What Comes Next?

As we look ahead, it's becoming clear that our understanding of interoception—and its profound impact on everyday life—is only beginning to unfold. What researchers are discovering reveals something quietly powerful and deeply healing, yet something that has also always been part of us. Interoception isn't just a term used in neuroscience labs or therapy offices; it belongs to everyone. It's an intrinsic aspect of being human.

When we start tuning into the body, even in small ways, meaningful shifts can occur. Many challenges people face, both mental and physical, aren't happening only "in the mind." They are held in the body, showing up as tight chests, racing hearts, fatigue, numbness, unsettled stomachs, or a vague sense that something is off. Interoceptive awareness offers a different way to relate to these experiences. Instead of pushing through, judging, or trying to silence the body, we can begin to listen. When we do, sensations become information rather than problems.

Because so much information is carried in the body, listening inward supports change across many areas of life. It helps us notice early signs of stress, hunger, or overload before they escalate. It enhances emotional understanding by helping us recognize feelings as they arise in the body, making us less reactive and more able to respond with steadiness. And because our thoughts are continually influenced by bodily states, greater mind–body awareness leads to clearer, more balanced decisions. Eventually, this kind of listening fosters a more grounded sense of self, one anchored from within rather than primarily shaped by external pressures. In relationships, recognizing our own internal signals makes it easier to meet others with empathy, compassion, and a sense of safety.

One of the most encouraging aspects of interoception is how simple it is to access. Learning to notice your breath, feel tension, identify internal cues, or respond with care doesn't need special tools, medication, or even a therapist. These everyday skills can be practiced anywhere and woven into ordinary moments of life. That accessibility matters. It puts control back in our hands and reminds us that healing doesn't always begin with fixing something broken. Often, it begins with noticing what's already working.

This shift in listening also has the potential to transform how care is delivered on a larger scale. When we recognize that many struggles follow common patterns in the body, treatment becomes less fragmented and more compassionate. Therapy no longer needs to choose between body or mind—it can work with both, from the inside out and the outside in. Bottom-up approaches that promote regulation, safety, and grounding create space for insight, while top-down methods help interpret feelings and offer options for change. Rather than competing, these approaches complement one another. In this kind of care, the priority shifts from just reducing symptoms to building capacity, supporting regulation, and catching overwhelm early before it becomes a crisis. Over time, mind–body care may feel less like a specialized method and more like a natural standard for supporting whole people.

For some, learning about interoception brings clarity and relief, giving words to experiences they've always felt and practical ways to support their nervous systems in daily life. For others, turning toward the body may feel new or even uncomfortable, especially if bodily cues have long been linked to distress. If that's the case, it's important to understand that healing isn't about forcing awareness. It's about moving gently, at your own pace, with choice and support. The body gradually learns safety, and that process can be deeply healing.

As our understanding of interoception deepens, it's possible to imagine a world where more people feel grounded and settled, better able to connect with themselves and with others—where there is enough energy not only to move through daily life but also to enjoy it. I look forward to a time when conversations about interoception no longer require explanation because listening to the body is simply understood as part of well-being.

Writing this book has been an act of hope—hope for a world with greater well-being, one that's kinder and less reactive, where self-judgment softens into curiosity, and bodies are seen as partners rather than problems. My wish is that these pages have offered not only insight but also permission—to listen more closely, respond more gently, and trust the wisdom that has always been there. May interoception continue to open doors to deeper connection with yourself, shaping not just how we heal, but how we live.

# Notes

## Chapter 1: Understanding Interoception


1 Erik Ceunen, Johan W. S. Vlaeyen, and Ilse Van Diest, "On the Origin of Interoception," *Frontiers in Psychology* 7 (May 2016): 743, https://doi.org/10.3389/fpsyg.2016.00743.

2 Bruce H. Friedman, "Feelings and the Body: The Jamesian Perspective on Autonomic Specificity of Emotion," *Biological Psychology* 84, no. 3 (2010): 384, https://doi.org/10.1016/j.biopsycho.2009.10.006.

3 Antoine Bechara and Antonio R. Damasio, "The Somatic Marker Hypothesis: A Neural Theory of Economic Decision," *Games and Economic Behavior* 52, no. 2 (2005): 339, https://doi.org/10.1016/j.geb.2004.06.010.

4 A. D. (Bud) Craig, *How Do You Feel?: An Interoceptive Moment with Your Neurobiological Self* (Princeton University Press, 2014), 4.

5 Antonio Damasio, *Descartes' Error: Emotion, Reason, and the Human Brain* (Penguin Books, 2005).

6 Nikolas Heim, Marina Bobou, Michal Tanzer, Paul M. Jenkinson, Christiane Steinert, and Aikaterini Fotopoulou, "Psychological Interventions for Interoception in Mental Health Disorders: A Systematic Review of Randomized-Controlled Trials," *Psychiatry and Clinical Neurosciences* 77, no. 10 (2023): 530, https://doi.org/10.1111/pcn.13576.

7 Thomas Ritz, André Schulz, and Sahib Khalsa, "The Golden Age of Integrative Neuroscience? The Brain Joins the Body in the Latest Renaissance of Interoception Research," *Biological Psychology* 192 (October 2024): 108851, https://doi.org/10.1016/j.biopsycho.2024.108851.


## Chapter 2: The Science of Interoception


1 Sahib S. Khalsa and Rachel C. Lapidus, "Can Interoception Improve the Pragmatic Search for Biomarkers in Psychiatry?," *Frontiers in Psychiatry* 7 (July 2016): 121, https://doi.org/10.3389/fpsyt.2016.00121; Swarna Buddha Nayok, Vanteemar S. Sreeraj, Venkataram Shivakumar, and Ganesan Venkatasubramanian, "A Primer on Interoception and Its Importance in Psychiatry," *Clinical Psychopharmacology and Neuroscience* 21, no. 2 (2023): 252–61, https://doi.org/10.9758/cpn.2023.21.2.252.

2 Paul Grossman, "Respiratory Sinus Arrhythmia (RSA), Vagal Tone and Biobehavioral Integration: Beyond Parasympathetic Function," *Biological Psychology* 186 (February 2024): 108739, https://doi.org/10.1016/j.biopsycho.2023.108739.

3 Li Ma, Han-Bing Wang, and Kenji Hashimoto, "The Vagus Nerve: An Old but New Player in Brain–Body Communication," *Brain, Behavior, and Immunity* 124 (February 2025): 28–39, https://doi.org/10.1016/j.bbi.2024.11.023.

4 Ma et al., "Vagus Nerve."

5 Ma et al., "Vagus Nerve."

6 Ruohan Zhang, Hanfei Deng, and Xiong Xiao, "The Insular Cortex: An Interface Between Sensation, Emotion, and Cognition," *Neuroscience Bulletin* 40 (May 2024): 1766, https://doi.org/10.1007/s12264-024-01211-4.

7 A. D. (Bud) Craig, *How Do You Feel?: An Interoceptive Moment with Your Neurobiological Self* (Princeton University Press, 2014), 45.
8 Craig, *How Do You Feel?*, 223.
9 Craig, *How Do You Feel?*, 254.
10 Zhang et al., "Insular Cortex," 1763.
11 Robert M. Sapolsky, *Why Zebras Don't Get Ulcers: The Acclaimed Guide to Stress, Stress-Related Diseases, and Coping*, 3rd ed. (St. Martin's Press, 2004).
12 Julian F. Thayer and Richard D. Lane, "A Model of Neurovisceral Integration in Emotion Regulation and Dysregulation," *Journal of Affective Disorders* 61, no. 3 (2000): 201–16, https://doi.org/10.1016/S0165-0327(00)00338-4.
13 Kasia Kozlowska, Peter Walker, Loyola McLean, and Pascal Carrive, "Fear and the Defense Cascade: Clinical Implications and Management," *Harvard Review of Psychiatry* 23, no. 4 (2015): 263–87, https://doi.org/10.1097/HRP.0000000000000065.
14 Lisa Feldman Barrett and Karen Quigley, "Interoception: The Secret Ingredient," *Cerebrum*, July 1, 2021, https://pmc.ncbi.nlm.nih.gov/articles/PMC8493823.
15 Barrett and Quigley, "Interoception."

## Chapter 3: Interoception in Daily Life

1 Dannyelle Valente, Anne Theurel, and Edouard Gentaz, "The Role of Visual Experience in the Production of Emotional Facial Expressions by Blind People: A Review," *Psychonomic Bulletin and Review* 25 (June 2017): 483, https://doi.org/10.3758/s13423-017-1338-0.
2 Beate M. Herbert, Olga Pollatos, and Rainer Schandry, "Interoceptive Sensitivity and Emotion Processing: An EEG Study," *International Journal of Psychophysiology* 65, no. 3 (2007): 214, https://doi.org/10.1016/j.ijpsycho.2007.04.007.
3 Antonio Damasio, *Descartes' Error: Emotion, Reason, and the Human Brain* (Penguin Books, 2005).
4 Damasio, *Descartes' Error.*
5 A. D. (Bud) Craig, *How Do You Feel?: An Interoceptive Moment with Your Neurobiological Self* (Princeton University Press, 2014).
6 Craig, *How Do You Feel?*
7 Antonio Damasio, *Self Comes to Mind: Constructing the Conscious Brain* (Vintage Books, 2012).
8 Norman A. S. Farb, Zindel V. Segal, Helen Mayberg, Jim Bean, Deborah McKeon, Zainab Fatima, et al., "Attending to the Present: Mindfulness Meditation Reveals Distinct Neural Modes of Self-Reference," *Social Cognitive and Affective Neuroscience* 2, no. 4 (2007): 313–22, https://doi.org/10.1093/scan/nsm030.
9 Craig, *How Do You Feel?*, 6.
10 Nikolas Heim, Marina Bobou, Michal Tanzer, Paul M. Jenkinson, Christiane Steinert, and Aikaterini Fotopoulou, "Psychological Interventions for Interoception in Mental Health Disorders: A Systematic Review of Randomized-Controlled Trials," *Psychiatry and Clinical Neurosciences* 77, no. 10 (2023): 530, https://doi.org/10.1111/pcn.13576.
11 Sahib S. Khalsa and Rachel C. Lapidus, "Can Interoception Improve the Pragmatic Search for Biomarkers in Psychiatry?," *Frontiers in Psychiatry* 7 (July 2016): 121, https://doi.org/10.3389/fpsyt.2016.00121.
12 Heim et al., "Psychological Interventions," 530.

## Chapter 4: How Interoception Is Measured

1 Rebecca Brewer, Jennifer Murphy, and Geoffrey Bird, "Atypical Interoception as a Common Risk Factor for Psychopathology: A Review," *Neuroscience and Biobehavioral Reviews* 130 (November 2021): 472, https://doi.org/10.1016/j.neubiorev.2021.07.036.

2 Felix A. Schoeller, Ben Zhang, Teresa Garcia, and Nicco Reggente, "There Is No Such Thing as Interoception," *Frontiers in Psychology* 16 (February 2025): 1488415, https://doi.org/10.3389/fpsyg.2025.1488415.

3 Olivier Desmedt, Olivier Luminet, Marta Walentynowicz, and Olivier Corneille, "The New Measures of Interoceptive Accuracy: A Systematic Review and Assessment," *Neuroscience and Biobehavioral Reviews* 153 (October 2023): 105388, https://doi.org/10.1016/j.neubiorev.2023.105388.

4 Wolf E. Mehling, Michael Acree, Anita Stewart, Jonathan Silas, and Alexander Jones, "The Multidimensional Assessment of Interoceptive Awareness, Version 2 (MAIA-2)," *PLOS ONE* 13, no. 12 (2018): e0208034, https://doi.org/10.1371/journal.pone.0208034.

5 Desmedt et al., "New Measures of Interoceptive Accuracy," 37–38.

6 Chatrin Suksasilp and Sarah N. Garfinkel, "Towards a Comprehensive Assessment of Interoception in a Multi-Dimensional Framework," *Biological Psychology* 168 (February 2022): 108262, https://doi.org/10.1016/j.biopsycho.2022.108262.

7 William Bruce Cameron, *Informal Sociology: A Casual Introduction to Sociological Thinking* (Random House, 1964), 13, https://archive.org/details/informalsociolog0000came/page/n5/mode/2up?view=theater.

8 Mehling et al., "Multidimensional Assessment of Interoceptive Awareness"; Wolf E. Mehling, *Multidimensional Assessment of Interoceptive Awareness (MAIA) Version 2* (University of California, San Francisco, 2018), https://osher.ucsf.edu/sites/osher.ucsf.edu/files/inline-files/MAIA2%202018.05.27.pdf.

## Chapter 5: Miscommunication Between Body and Brain

1 Larissa Medeiros Leão, Amalia Cinthia Meneses Rêgo, and Irami Araújo-Filho, "Interoception: Current Knowledge Gaps and Future Directions in Neuroscience, Psychopathology, and Clinical Applications," *International Journal of Innovative Research in Medical Science* 10, no. 3 (2025): 104–5, https://doi.org/10.23958/ijirms/vol10-i03/2041.

2 Leão et al., "Interoception," 104–5.

3 Leão et al., "Interoception," 104–5.

4 Kelly Mahler, Kerri Hample, Claudia Jones, Joseph Sensenig, Phoebe Thomasco, and Claudia Hilton, "Impact of an Interoception-Based Program on Emotion Regulation in Autistic Children," *Occupational Therapy International*, April 20, 2022, https://doi.org/10.1155/2022/9328967.

5 Leão et al., "Interoception," 104.

6 Alisha M. Bruton, Laura Levy, Navdeep Kaur Rai, Dana Dharmakaya Colgan, and Jeanette M. Johnstone, "Diminished Interoceptive Accuracy in Attention-Deficit/Hyperactivity Disorder: A Systematic Review," *Psychophysiology* 62, no. 2 (2025): e14750, https://doi.org/10.1111/psyp.14750.

7 Austin M. Matus, Barbara Riegel, and Michael R. Rickels, "Interoceptive Awareness Is Associated with Impaired Awareness of Hypoglycemia in Adults with Type 1 Diabetes," *Diabetes Care* 48, no. 1 (2025): 103, https://doi.org/10.2337/dc24-1720.

8 Christopher Burton, Helen Dawes, Simon Goodwill, Michael Thelwell, and Caroline Dalton, "Within and Between-Day Variation and Associations of Symptoms in Long Covid: Intensive Longitudinal Study," *PLOS ONE* 18, no. 1 (2023): 2, e0280343, https://doi.org/10.1371/journal.pone.0280343.
9 Brian S. Kim and David Artis, "The Sensory Neuroimmune Frontier," *Immunity* 58, no. 5 (2025): 1036, https://doi.org/10.1016/j.immuni.2025.03.018.
10 R. A. Hauser, D. Matias, and B. Rawlings, "The Ligamentous Cervical Instability Etiology of Human Disease from the Forward Head-Facedown Lifestyle: Emphasis on Obstruction of Fluid Flow into and out of the Brain," *Frontiers in Neurology* 15 (November 2024): 1430390, https://doi.org/10.3389/fneur.2024.1430390.
11 Michael Ganci, Emra Suleyman, Henry Butt, and Michelle Ball, "The Role of the Brain–Gut–Microbiota Axis in Psychology: The Importance of Considering Gut Microbiota in the Development, Perpetuation, and Treatment of Psychological Disorders," *Brain and Behavior* 9, no. 11 (2019): e01408, https://doi.org/10.1002/brb3.1408.
12 Leon M. T. Dicks, "Gut Bacteria and Neurotransmitters," *Microorganisms* 10, no. 9 (2022): 1838, https://doi.org/10.3390/microorganisms10091838.
13 Baoli Zhu et al., "Human Gut Microbiome: The Second Genome of Human Body," *Protein & Cell* 1 (2010): 718, https://doi.org/10.1007/s13238-010-0093-z.
14 Jake Robinson, *Invisible Friends: How Microbes Shape Our Lives and the World Around Us* (Pelagic Publishing, 2023).
15 Ganci et al., "Role of the Brain–Gut–Microbiota Axis."
16 Ganci et al., "Role of the Brain–Gut–Microbiota Axis."

## Chapter 6: How Thoughts Shape Interoception

1 "The Nocebo Effect: History and Contemporary Applications," Mayo Clinic, February 16, 2024, https://mcpress.mayoclinic.org/research-innovation/the-nocebo-effect-history-contemporary-applications.
2 Nayla M. Khoury, Jacqueline Lutz, and Zev Schuman-Olivier, "Interoception in Psychiatric Disorders: A Review of Randomized, Controlled Trials with Interoception-Based Interventions," *Harvard Review of Psychiatry* 26, no. 5 (2018): 250–63, https://doi.org/10.1097/hrp.0000000000000170.
3 Lisa Feldman Barrett and W. Kyle Simmons, "Interoceptive Predictions in the Brain," *Nature Reviews Neuroscience* 16 (May 2015): 419, https://doi.org/10.1038/nrn3950.
4 Dana Dharmakaya Colgan, Ashley Eddy, Kaylie Green, and Barry Oken, "Adaptive Body Awareness Predicts Fewer Central Sensitization–Related Symptoms and Explains Relationship Between Central Sensitization–Related Symptoms and Pain Intensity: A Cross-Sectional Study Among Individuals with Chronic Pain," *Pain Practice* 22, no. 2 (2022): 223, https://doi.org/10.1111/papr.13083; Lucy Snell, Katie Bannister, Yeetung Hong, Matthew Garner, Gaby Pfeifer, and Jayne Morriss, "The Relationship Between Interoception and Anxiety Disorders in Adult Clinical Populations—A Systematic Review and Narrative Synthesis," preprint, PsyArXiv, June 24, 2025, 28, https://doi.org/10.31234/osf.io/7b3v9_v1.
5 Randy A. Sansone and Lori A. Sansone, "Rumination: Relationships with Physical Health," *Innovations in Clinical Neuroscience* 9, no. 2 (2012): 29–34, https://psycnet.apa.org/record/2012-06960-004.
6 Lisa Feldman Barrett and Karen Quigley, "Interoception: The Secret Ingredient," *Cerebrum*, July 1, 2021, https://pmc.ncbi.nlm.nih.gov/articles/PMC8493823.

## Chapter 7: The Influence of Early Attachments

1 "These Amazing Animal Moms Adopted Orphans as Their Own," IFAW, March 8, 2024, www.ifaw.org/journal/amazing-animal-moms-adopted-orphans.
2 Allan N. Schore, *Affect Regulation and the Origin of the Self: The Neurobiology of Emotional Development* (Routledge, 2015).
3 Jeffry A. Simpson and W. Steven Rholes, "Adult Attachment, Stress, and Romantic Relationships," *Current Opinion in Psychology* 13 (February 2017): 19, https://doi.org/10.1016/j.copsyc.2016.04.006.
4 Susan Hart, *The Impact of Attachment: Developmental Neuroaffective Psychology* (Norton, 2011), 23.
5 Hart, *Impact of Attachment,* 153.
6 Kristina Oldroyd, Monisha Pasupathi, and Cecilia Wainryb, "Social Antecedents to the Development of Interoception: Attachment Related Processes Are Associated with Interoception," *Frontiers in Psychology* 10 (April 2019): 712, https://doi.org/10.3389/fpsyg.2019.00712.
7 Hart, *Impact of Attachment,* 62.
8 Oldroyd et al., "Social Antecedents."
9 Oldroyd et al., "Social Antecedents."
10 Daniel J. Siegel and Mary Hartzell, *Parenting from the Inside Out* (Scribe Publications, 2014), 87.
11 Oldroyd et al., "Social Antecedents."
12 Andrew Arnold, "Some Body to Love: Intrapersonal and Interoceptive Components of Social Connection" (PhD diss., University of California, San Diego, 2022), 16, https://escholarship.org/content/qt47k8b3jc/qt47k8b3jc.pdf.
13 Lorenzo Lucherini Angeletti, Emanuele Cassioli, Livio Tarchi, Cristiano Dani, Marco Faldi, Rachele Martini, et al., "From Early Relational Experiences to Non-Suicidal Self-Injury in Anorexia and Bulimia Nervosa: A Structural Equation Model Unraveling the Role of Impairments in Interoception," *Eating and Weight Disorders* 29, no. 22 (2024): 8, https://doi.org/10.1007/s40519-024-01651-x.
14 Angeletti et al., "Early Relational Experiences," 8.
15 Oldroyd et al., "Social Antecedents."
16 Oldroyd et al., "Social Antecedents."
17 Jonathan Gibson, "Trauma, Early Life Stress, and Mindfulness in Adulthood," *BMC Psychology* 12, no. 71 (2024): 5–6, https://doi.org/10.1186/s40359-024-01563-6.
18 Oldroyd et al., "Social Antecedents."
19 Oldroyd et al., "Social Antecedents."

## Chapter 8: Understanding the Stress Response

1 Robert M. Sapolsky, *Why Zebras Don't Get Ulcers: The Acclaimed Guide to Stress, Stress-Related Diseases, and Coping,* 3rd ed. (St. Martin's Press, 2004), 2.
2 Sapolsky, *Why Zebras Don't Get Ulcers.*
3 André Schulz and Claus Vögele, "Interoception and Stress," *Frontiers in Psychology* 6 (July 2015): 993, https://doi.org/10.3389/fpsyg.2015.00993.
4 Roberta A. Allegretta, Katia Rovelli, and Michela Balconi, "The Role of Emotion Regulation and Awareness in Psychosocial Stress: An EEG-Psychometric Correlational Study," *Healthcare* 12, no. 15 (2024): 1491, https://doi.org/10.3390/healthcare12151491.

5 Philippe R. Goldin, Kateri McRae, Wiveka Ramel, and James J. Gross, "The Neural Bases of Emotion Regulation: Reappraisal and Suppression of Negative Emotion," *Biological Psychiatry* 63, no. 9 (2008): 578–84, https://doi.org/10.1016/j.biopsych.2007.05.031.

## Chapter 9: Trauma Symptoms and Interoceptive Interruptions

1 American Psychiatric Association, *Quick Reference to the Diagnostic Criteria from DSM-III* (American Psychiatric Association, 1980), 137.

2 C. Benjet, E. Bromet, E. G. Karam, R. C. Kessler, K. A. McLaughlin, A. M. Ruscio, et al., "The Epidemiology of Traumatic Event Exposure Worldwide: Results from the World Mental Health Survey Consortium," *Psychological Medicine* 46, no. 2 (2015): 328, https://doi.org/10.1017/s0033291715001981.

3 Vincent J. Felitti, Robert F. Anda, Dale Nordenberg, Valerie Edwards, Mary P. Koss, James S. Marks, et al., "Relationship of Childhood Abuse and Household Dysfunction to Many of the Leading Causes of Death in Adults: The Adverse Childhood Experiences (ACE) Study," *American Journal of Preventive Medicine* 14, no. 4 (1998): 245–58, https://doi.org/10.1016/s0749-3797(98)00017-8.

4 Bessel van der Kolk, "Psychiatry Must Stop Ignoring Trauma," posted February 2, 2015, by BigThink, YouTube, 4 min., 3 sec., www.youtube.com/watch?v=HR22lvBo1rQ.

5 Nikolas Heim, Marina Bobou, Michal Tanzer, Paul M. Jenkinson, Christiane Steinert, and Aikaterini Fotopoulou, "Psychological Interventions for Interoception in Mental Health Disorders: A Systematic Review of Randomized-Controlled Trials," *Psychiatry and Clinical Neurosciences* 77, no. 10 (2023): 530, https://doi.org/10.1111/pcn.13576; Negar Fani, Travis Fulton, and Boris Botzanowski, "The Neurophysiology of Interoceptive Disruptions in Trauma-Exposed Populations," in *Current Topics in Behavioral Neurosciences*, ed. Bart A. Ellenbroek, Martin P. Paulus, Jocelien Olivier, and Katrin H. Preller, vol. 74, *Perceptual Dysregulation in Psychiatric Nosology*, ed. Sahib Khalsa and Albert Powers (Springer, 2024), 2, https://doi.org/10.1007/7854_2024_469.

6 Breanne E. Kearney and Ruth A. Lanius, "The Brain-Body Disconnect: A Somatic Sensory Basis for Trauma-Related Disorders," *Frontiers in Neuroscience* 16 (November 2022): 1015749, https://doi.org/10.3389/fnins.2022.1015749.

7 Kelly Leech, "The Felt Sense of the Body: An Empirical Evaluation of a Mindful-Interoceptive Approach to Post-Traumatic Stress Disorder" (PhD diss., Bond University, 2024), 28, https://pure.bond.edu.au/ws/portalfiles/portal/249229624/Kelly_Leech_Thesis.pdf.

8 Bessel van der Kolk, "The Body Keeps the Score: Approaches to the Psychobiology of Posttraumatic Stress Disorder," in *Traumatic Stress: The Effects of Overwhelming Experience on Mind, Body, and Society*, ed. Bessel van der Kolk, Alexander McFarlane, and Lars Weisæth (Guilford Press, 2008), 218–19.

9 John Briere and Joseph Spinazzola, "Phenomenology and Psychological Assessment of Complex Posttraumatic States," *Journal of Traumatic Stress* 18, no. 5 (2005): 403, https://doi.org/10.1002/jts.20048.

10 Gabor Maté, *In the Realm of Hungry Ghosts: Close Encounters with Addiction* (North Atlantic Books, 2010), 36.

11 Leech, "Felt Sense," 45.

12 Peter A. Levine, *In an Unspoken Voice: How the Body Releases Trauma and Restores Goodness* (North Atlantic Books, 2010), 136.

13 Levine, *In an Unspoken Voice*, 136.

## Chapter 10: Trauma and the Disrupted Sense of Self

1 Peter A. Levine, *In an Unspoken Voice: How the Body Releases Trauma and Restores Goodness* (North Atlantic Books, 2010), 137.

2 Bessel van der Kolk, *The Body Keeps the Score: Brain, Mind, and Body in the Healing of Trauma* (Viking, 2014), 99.

3 Niloofar Afari, Sandra Ahumada, Lisa Johnson Wright, Sheeva Mostoufi, Golnaz Golnari, Veronica Reis, et al., "Psychological Trauma and Functional Somatic Syndromes," *Psychosomatic Medicine* 76, no. 1 (2014): 2, https://doi.org/10.1097/psy.0000000000000010.

4 Ruth A. Lanius, Braeden A. Terpou, and Margaret C. McKinnon, "The Sense of Self in the Aftermath of Trauma: Lessons from the Default Mode Network in Posttraumatic Stress Disorder," *European Journal of Psychotraumatology* 11, no. 1 (2020): 1807703, https://doi.org/10.1080/20008198.2020.1807703.

5 Cindy van Sleeuwen, Mirjam van Zuiden, Saskia B. J. Koch, Jessie L. Frijling, Dick J. Veltman, Miranda Olff, et al., "How Does It Feel? An Exploration of Neurobiological and Clinical Correlates of Alexithymia in Trauma-Exposed Police-Officers with and without PTSD," *European Journal of Psychotraumatology* 14, no. 2 (2023): 2281187, https://doi.org/10.1080/20008066.2023.2281187.

6 Rebecca Brewer, Jennifer Murphy, and Geoffrey Bird, "Atypical Interoception as a Common Risk Factor for Psychopathology: A Review," *Neuroscience and Biobehavioral Reviews* 130 (November 2021): 480, https://doi.org/10.1016/j.neubiorev.2021.07.036.

7 Isabella K. Ferraro and Amanda M. Taylor, "Adult Attachment Styles and Emotional Regulation: The Role of Interoceptive Awareness and Alexithymia," *Personality and Individual Differences* 173 (April 2021): 110641, https://doi.org/10.1016/j.paid.2021.110641.

8 Van der Kolk, *The Body Keeps the Score*, 98.

## Chapter 11: Common Threads, Synergistic Impacts, and Unintended Consequences

1 "Mental Disorders," *World Health Organization,* updated September 30, 2025, www.who.int/news-room/fact-sheets/detail/mental-disorders.

2 Substance Abuse and Mental Health Services Administration, *Key Substance Use and Mental Health Indicators in the United States: Results from the 2024 National Survey on Drug Use and Health* (Center for Behavioral Health Statistics and Quality, 2025), 32, www.samhsa.gov/data/sites/default/files/reports/rpt56287/2024-nsduh-annual-national-report.pdf.

3 *Global Status Report on Alcohol and Health and Treatment of Substance Use Disorders* (World Health Organization, 2024), iv, https://iris.who.int/server/api/core/bitstreams/32b161e9-5683-40f5-a1c3-1c92a76d5cda/content.

4 Catharina J. Candussi, Russell Kabir, and Madhini Sivasubramanian, "Problematic Smartphone Usage, Prevalence, and Patterns Among University Students: A Systematic Review," *Journal of Affective Disorders Reports* 14 (December 2023): 100643, https://doi.org/10.1016/j.jadr.2023.100643.

5 *Suicide Worldwide in 2021: Global Health Estimates* (World Health Organization, 2025), 1, www.who.int/publications/i/item/9789240110069.
6 Substance Abuse and Mental Health Services Administration, *Key Substance Use and Mental Health Indicators*, 38.
7 Ellen-ge Denton and Kiara Álvarez, "The Global Prevalence of Nonsuicidal Self-Injury Among Adolescents," *JAMA Network Open* 7, no. 6 (2024): e2415406, https://doi.org/10.1001/jamanetworkopen.2024.15406.
8 Gabriel A. Benavidez, Whitney E. Zahnd, Peiyin Hung, and Jan M. Eberth, "Chronic Disease Prevalence in the US: Sociodemographic and Geographic Variations by ZIP Code Tabulation Area," *Preventing Chronic Disease* 21 (February 2024): 230267, https://doi.org/10.5888/pcd21.230267.
9 Gallup and Meta, *The Global State of Social Connections* (Gallup, 2023), 2, www.gallup.com/analytics/509675/state-of-social-connections.aspx.
10 Martina Saltafossi, Detlef Heck, Daniel S. Kluger, and Somogy Varga, "Common Threads: Altered Interoceptive Processes Across Affective and Anxiety Disorders," *Journal of Affective Disorders* 369 (January 2025): 244, https://doi.org/10.1016/j.jad.2024.09.135.
11 Saltafossi et al., "Common Threads," 246.
12 Rebecca Brewer, Jennifer Murphy, and Geoffrey Bird, "Atypical Interoception as a Common Risk Factor for Psychopathology: A Review," *Neuroscience and Biobehavioral Reviews* 130 (November 2021): 471, https://doi.org/10.1016/j.neubiorev.2021.07.036.
13 Mario Mikulincer, Phillip R. Shaver, and Zahava Solomon, "An Attachment Perspective on Traumatic and Posttraumatic Reactions," in *Attachment Theory and Research: New Directions and Emerging Themes*, ed. Jeffry A. Simpson and W. Steven Rholes (Guilford Press, 2015).
14 Vincent J. Felitti, Robert F. Anda, Dale Nordenberg, Valerie Edwards, Mary P. Koss, James S. Marks, et al., "Relationship of Childhood Abuse and Household Dysfunction to Many of the Leading Causes of Death in Adults: The Adverse Childhood Experiences (ACE) Study," *American Journal of Preventive Medicine* 14, no. 4 (1998): 245, https://doi.org/10.1016/s0749-3797(98)00017-8.
15 Han Shi Chew, Rou Yi Soong, Wei How Darryl Ang, Jia Wen Ngooi, Jiyoung Park, Jenna Qing Yun Ow Yong, et al., "The Global Prevalence of Emotional Eating in Overweight and Obese Populations: A Systematic Review and Meta-Analysis," *British Journal of Psychology* 116, no. 2 (2025): 484, https://doi.org/10.1111/bjop.12768.
16 Clémence Willem, Marie-Charlotte Gandolphe, Méline Roussel, Hélène Verkindt, François Pattou, and Jean-Louis Nandrino, "Difficulties in Emotion Regulation and Deficits in Interoceptive Awareness in Moderate and Severe Obesity," *Eating and Weight Disorders—Studies on Anorexia, Bulimia and Obesity* 24 (2019): 633–44, https://doi.org/10.1007/s40519-019-00738-0.
17 Antonios Dakanalis, Maria Mentzelou, Souzana K. Papadopoulou, Dimitrios Papandreou, Maria Spanoudaki, Georgios K. Vasios, et al., "The Association of Emotional Eating with Overweight/Obesity, Depression, Anxiety/Stress, and Dietary Patterns: A Review of the Current Clinical Evidence," *Nutrients* 15, no. 5 (2023): 1173, https://doi.org/10.3390/nu15051173.

## Chapter 12: Anxiety Disorders

1 "Anxiety Disorders," World Health Organization, September 8, 2025, www.who.int/news-room/fact-sheets/detail/anxiety-disorders.

2 Huiru Cao, Yang Wu, Hui Yin, Yanqi Sun, Hui Yuan, and Mengjun Tao, "Global Trends in the Incidence of Anxiety Disorders from 1990 to 2019: Joinpoint and Age-Period-Cohort Analysis Study," *JMIR Public Health and Surveillance* 10 (January 2024): e49609, https://doi.org/10.2196/49609.

3 Kristin L. Szuhany and Naomi M. Simon, "Anxiety Disorders: A Review," *JAMA* 328, no. 24 (2022): 2431–32, https://doi.org/10.1001/jama.2022.22744.

4 Lucy Snell, Katie Bannister, Yeetung Hong, Matthew Garner, Gaby Pfeifer, and Jayne Morriss, "The Relationship Between Interoception and Anxiety Disorders in Adult Clinical Populations—A Systematic Review and Narrative Synthesis," preprint, PsyArXiv, June 24, 2025, 28, https://doi.org/10.31234/osf.io/7b3v9_v1.

5 I. Schmalbach and K. Petrowski, "The Role of Interoceptive Awareness in Social Anxiety Disorder—Results of an Internet-Based CBT-Manualized Therapist Delivered Group-Treatment," *BMC Psychology* 13, no. 742 (2025): 2, https://doi.org/10.1186/s40359-025-03013-3.

6 Carolin Lea Wolters, "'I Don't Want to Miss a Symptom'—The Role of Biased Interoception in Somatic Symptoms and Illness Anxiety" (PhD diss., University of Cologne, 2023), 5, 7, https://kups.ub.uni-koeln.de/71113/1/Dissertation%20Carolin%20Wolters%2009_2023.pdf.

7 Hannah S. Savage and Sarah Garfinkel, "Making Sense of Sensation: A Model of Interoceptive Attribution and Appraisal with Clinical Applications," preprint, PsyArXiv, July 11, 2025, 6–7, https://doi.org/10.31234/osf.io/bsma9_v1.

8 Savage and Garfinkel, "Making Sense of Sensation," 7.

9 Schmalbach and Petrowski, "Role of Interoceptive Awareness," 2.

10 S. Krautwurst, A. L. Gerlach, and M. Witthöft, "Interoception in Pathological Health Anxiety," *Journal of Abnormal Psychology* 125, no. 8 (2016): 1179, https://doi.org/10.1037/abn0000210.

11 Harry Man Xiong Lai, Michelle Cleary, Thiagarajan Sitharthan, and Glenn E. Hunt, "Prevalence of Comorbid Substance Use, Anxiety and Mood Disorders in Epidemiological Surveys, 1990–2014: A Systematic Review and Meta-Analysis," *Drug and Alcohol Dependence* 154 (September 2015): 1, https://doi.org/10.1016/j.drugalcdep.2015.05.031.

12 Kathleen T. Brady, Louise F. Haynes, Karen J. Hartwell, and Therese K. Killeen, "Substance Use Disorders and Anxiety: A Treatment Challenge for Social Workers," *Social Work in Public Health* 28, no. 3–4 (2013): 407–23, https://doi.org/10.1080/19371918.2013.774675.

13 Julia Y. Gorday and Joseph R. Bardeen, "Problematic Smartphone Use Influences the Relationship Between Experiential Avoidance and Anxiety," *Cyberpsychology, Behavior, and Social Networking* 25, no. 1 (2022): 72, https://doi.org/10.1089/cyber.2021.0062.

14 Natasha Kim de Oliveira da Fonseca, Marianna de Abreu Costa, Natan Pereira Gosmann, Roberta Dalle Molle, Francine Guimarães Gonçalves, Alice Cardozo Silva, et al., "Emotional Eating in Women with Generalized Anxiety Disorder," *Trends in Psychiatry and Psychotherapy* 45 (October 2023): 1–9, https://doi.org/10.47626/2237-6089-2021-0399.

15 Ryan J. Lackner and David M. Fresco, "Interaction Effect of Brooding Rumination and Interoceptive Awareness on Depression and Anxiety Symptoms," *Behaviour Research and Therapy* 85 (October 2016): 43–52, https://doi.org/10.1016/j.brat.2016.08.007.

16 Caroline Schlinkert, Beate M. Herbert, Nicola Baumann, and Sander L. Koole, "Preoccupied with the Body: Mild Stress Amplifies the Relation Between Rumination and Interoception," *Cognition and Emotion* 34, no. 7 (2020): 1382–94, https://doi.org/10.1080/02699931.2020.1746242.

## Chapter 13: Depression

1 "'Depression: Let's Talk' Says WHO, as Depression Tops List of Causes of Ill Health," World Health Organization, March 30, 2017, www.who.int/news/item/30-03-2017--depression-let-s-talk-says-who-as-depression-tops-list-of-causes-of-ill-health.
2 Substance Abuse and Mental Health Services Administration, *Key Substance Use and Mental Health Indicators in the United States: Results from the 2024 National Survey on Drug Use and Health* (Center for Behavioral Health Statistics and Quality, 2025), 31, www.samhsa.gov/data/sites/default/files/reports/rpt56287/2024-nsduh-annual-national-report.pdf.
3 Jorge Arias-de la Torre, Gemma Vilagut, Amy Ronaldson, Antoni Serrano-Blanco, Vicente Martín, Michele Peters, et al., "Prevalence and Variability of Current Depressive Disorder in 27 European Countries: A Population-Based Study," *Lancet Public Health* 6, no. 10 (2021): e729–38, https://doi.org/10.1016/s2468-2667(21)00047-5.
4 Michael Eggart, Juan Valdés-Stauber, Bruno Müller-Oerlinghausen, and Martin Heinze, "Dysfunctional Self-Reported Interoception Predicts Residual Symptom Burden of Fatigue in Major Depressive Disorder: An Observational Study," *BMC Psychiatry* 23, no. 667 (2023): 2, https://doi.org/10.1186/s12888-023-05168-y.
5 Xinzhong Li, Jiahui Zhou, Min Wang, Chengmin Yang, and Guibo Sun, "Cardiovascular Disease and Depression: A Narrative Review," *Frontiers in Cardiovascular Medicine* 10 (November 2023): 1274595, https://doi.org/10.3389/fcvm.2023.1274595.
6 Chieh-Hsin Lee and Fabrizio Giuliani, "The Role of Inflammation in Depression and Fatigue," *Frontiers in Immunology* 10 (July 2019): 1696, https://doi.org/10.3389/fimmu.2019.01696.
7 Mark Nolan, Elena Roman, Anurag Nasa, Kirk J. Levins, Erik O'Hanlon, Veronica O'Keane, et al., "Hippocampal and Amygdalar Volume Changes in Major Depressive Disorder: A Targeted Review and Focus on Stress," *Chronic Stress* 4 (January 2020), https://doi.org/10.1177/2470547020944553.
8 Tingyu Zhao, Ting Liu, Lu Wang, Kaiqiang Xie, Hui Tang, and Mimi Tang, "Dysfunction of Neurotransmitter Metabolism Is Associated with the Severity of Depression in First-Diagnosed, Drug-Naïve Depressed Patients," *Journal of Affective Disorders* 349 (March 2024): 332–41, https://doi.org/10.1016/j.jad.2024.01.023.
9 Akash Kumar, Jhilam Pramanik, Nandani Goyal, Dimple Chauhan, Bhagavathi Sundaram Sivamaruthi, Bhupendra G. Prajapati, et al., "Gut Microbiota in Anxiety and Depression: Unveiling the Relationships and Management Options," *Pharmaceuticals* 16, no. 4 (2023): 565, https://doi.org/10.3390/ph16040565.
10 Michael Ganci, Emra Suleyman, Henry Butt, and Michelle Ball, "The Role of the Brain–Gut–Microbiota Axis in Psychology: The Importance of Considering Gut Microbiota in the Development, Perpetuation, and Treatment of Psychological Disorders," *Brain and Behavior* 9, no. 11 (2019): e01408, https://doi.org/10.1002/brb3.1408.
11 Leon M. T. Dicks, "Gut Bacteria and Neurotransmitters," *Microorganisms* 10, no. 9 (2022): 1838, https://doi.org/10.3390/microorganisms10091838.
12 Eggart et al., "Dysfunctional Self-Reported Interoception."
13 Eggart et al., "Dysfunctional Self-Reported Interoception."

14 American Psychiatric Association, *Diagnostic and Statistical Manual of Mental Disorders: DSM-5*, 5th ed. (American Psychiatric Publishing, 2013), 184.
15 Chantal Hampf, Maike Scherf-Clavel, Carolin Weiß, Catherina Klüpfel, Saskia Stonawski, Leif Hommers, et al., "Effects of Anxious Depression on Antidepressant Treatment Response," *International Journal of Molecular Sciences* 24, no. 24 (2023): 17128, https://doi.org/10.3390/ijms242417128.
16 Huang-Li Lin, Wei-Yang Lee, Chun-Hao Liu, Wei-Yu Chiang, Ya-Ting Hsu, Chin-Fu Hsiao, et al., "The Clinical Characteristics and Manifestation of Anxious Depression Among Patients with Major Depressive Disorders—Results from a Taiwan Multicenter Study," *Psychiatry Investigation* 21, no. 6 (2024): 570, https://doi.org/10.30773/pi.2023.0419.
17 Lin et al., "Clinical Characteristics and Manifestation," 562.
18 Rita Ioana Platona, Georgiana Albina Căiță, Florica Voiță-Mekeres, Alexandra Oana Peia, and Radu Virgil Enătescu, "The Impact of Psychiatric Comorbidities Associated with Depression: A Literature Review," *Medicine and Pharmacy Reports* 97, no. 2 (2024): 144, https://doi.org/10.15386/mpr-2700.
19 Madhukar H. Trivedi, Michael E. Thase, J. Sloan Manning, and Richard H. Weisler, "Utilizing the DSM-5 Anxious Distress Specifier to Develop Treatment Strategies for Patients with Major Depressive Disorder," *Journal of Clinical Psychiatry* 78, no. 9 (2017): 1352, https://doi.org/10.4088/jcp.ot17015ah1.
20 Platona et al., "Impact of Psychiatric Comorbidities," 145–46.
21 Michael Berk, Ole Köhler-Forsberg, Megan Turner, Brenda W.J.H. Penninx, Anna Wrobel, Joseph Firth, et al., "Comorbidity Between Major Depressive Disorder and Physical Diseases: A Comprehensive Review of Epidemiology, Mechanisms, and Management," *World Psychiatry* 22, no. 3 (2023): 368, https://doi.org/10.1002/wps.21110.
22 Eggart et al., "Dysfunctional Self-Reported Interoception," 6.
23 Paul M. Jenkinson and Susan L. Rossell, "Disturbed Interoception in Body Dysmorphic Disorder: A Framework for Future Research," *Australian and New Zealand Journal of Psychiatry* 58, no. 4 (2023): 303, https://doi.org/10.1177/00048674231215030.
24 Zahir Vally, Mai Helmy, and Louis Fourie, "The Association Between Depression and Addictive Social Media Use During the COVID-19 Pandemic: The Mediating Role of Sense of Control," *PLOS ONE* 18 (September 2023): e0291034, https://doi.org/10.1371/journal.pone.0291034.
25 Platona et al., "Impact of Psychiatric Comorbidities," 145.
26 Ryan J. Lackner and David M. Fresco, "Interaction Effect of Brooding Rumination and Interoceptive Awareness on Depression and Anxiety Symptoms," *Behaviour Research and Therapy* 85 (October 2016): 44, https://doi.org/10.1016/j.brat.2016.08.007.
27 Zev Schuman-Olivier, Richa Gawande, Timothy B. Creedon, Alexandra Comeau, Todd Griswold, Lydia B. Smith, et al., "Change Starts with the Body: Interoceptive Appreciation Mediates the Effect of Mindfulness Training on Behavior Change—An Effect Moderated by Depression Severity," *Psychiatry Research* 342 (December 2024): 116230, https://doi.org/10.1016/j.psychres.2024.116230.
28 Julie Dunne, Michael Flores, Richa Gawande, and Zev Schuman-Olivier, "Losing Trust in Body Sensations: Interoceptive Awareness and Depression Symptom Severity Among Primary Care Patients," *Journal of Affective Disorders* 282 (March 2021): 1216, https://doi.org/10.1016/j.jad.2020.12.092.

29 Dunne et al., "Losing Trust in Body Sensations."
30 Dunne et al., "Losing Trust in Body Sensations."

## Chapter 14: OCD and Related Disorders

1 American Psychiatric Association, *Diagnostic and Statistical Manual of Mental Disorders: DSM-5*, 5th ed. (American Psychiatric Publishing, 2013), 235.
2 Steffen Moritz, Stella Schmotz, Luca Hoyer, and Amitai Abramovitch, "Motives for Performing Body-Focused Repetitive Behaviors (BFRBs): Similarities to and Differences from Non-Suicidal Self-Injurious and Stereotypic Movement Behaviors," *Cognitive Therapy and Research* 48 (July 2024): 1248, https://doi.org/10.1007/s10608-024-10501-0.
3 American Psychiatric Association, *DSM-5*, 235.
4 Lizzie A. Wilson, Jessica Scarfo, Mikayla E. Jones, and Imogen C. Rehm, "The Relationship Between Sensory Phenomena and Interoception Across the Obsessive–Compulsive Spectrum: A Systematic Review," *BMC Psychiatry* 25, no. 162 (2025): 2, https://doi.org/10.1186/s12888-024-06441-4.
5 Wilson et al., "Relationship Between Sensory Phenomena and Interoception," 2.
6 Laura B. Bragdon, Goi Khia Eng, Amanda Belanger, Katherine A. Collins, and Emily R. Stern, "Interoception and Obsessive-Compulsive Disorder: A Review of Current Evidence and Future Directions," *Frontiers in Psychiatry* 12 (August 2021): 686482, https://doi.org/10.3389/fpsyt.2021.686482.
7 Bragdon et al., "Interoception and Obsessive-Compulsive Disorder."
8 Wilson et al., "Relationship Between Sensory Phenomena and Interoception," 6.
9 Bragdon et al., "Interoception and Obsessive-Compulsive Disorder."
10 Bragdon et al., "Interoception and Obsessive-Compulsive Disorder."
11 Bragdon et al., "Interoception and Obsessive-Compulsive Disorder."
12 Alexey Tolchinsky, George F. R. Ellis, Michael Levin, Šárka Kaňková, and Jeffrey S. Burgdorf, "Disgust as a Primary Emotional System and Its Clinical Relevance," *Frontiers in Psychology* 15 (August 2024): 1454774, https://doi.org/10.3389/fpsyg.2024.1454774.
13 Aaron J. Blashill, William Grunewald, Angela Fang, Eliza Davidson, and Sabine Wilhelm, "Conformity to Masculine Norms and Symptom Severity Among Men Diagnosed with Muscle Dysmorphia vs. Body Dysmorphic Disorder," *PLOS ONE* 15, no. 8 (2020): e0237651, https://doi.org/10.1371/journal.pone.0237651.
14 Blashill et al., "Conformity to Masculine Norms."
15 Paul M. Jenkinson and Susan L. Rossell, "Disturbed Interoception in Body Dysmorphic Disorder: A Framework for Future Research," *Australian and New Zealand Journal of Psychiatry* 58, no. 4 (2023): 303, https://doi.org/10.1177/00048674231215030.
16 Jenkinson and Rossell, "Disturbed Interoception."
17 Aimée Margarita Jacquemot and Rebecca Park, "The Role of Interoception in the Pathogenesis and Treatment of Anorexia Nervosa: A Narrative Review," *Frontiers in Psychiatry* 11 (April 2020): 281, https://doi.org/10.3389/fpsyt.2020.00281.
18 William Grunewald, Sammi Fogelberg, Walton Ferguson, Sarah Hines, Bailey Fortenberry, and April R. Smith, "Longitudinal Relationships Between Specific Domains of Interoception and Muscle Dysmorphia Symptoms," *Eating Behaviors* 48 (January 2023): 101686, https://doi.org/10.1016/j.eatbeh.2022.101686.
19 Blashill et al., "Conformity to Masculine Norms."

20 Annarosa Cipriano, Stefania Cella, and Paolo Cotrufo, "Nonsuicidal Self-Injury: A Systematic Review," *Frontiers in Psychology* 8 (November 2017): 1946, https://doi.org/10.3389/fpsyg.2017.01946.
21 Richard T. Liu, "The Epidemiology of Non-Suicidal Self-Injury: Lifetime Prevalence, Sociodemographic and Clinical Correlates, and Treatment Use in a Nationally Representative Sample of Adults in England," *Psychological Medicine* 53, no. 1 (2021): 274–82, https://doi.org/10.1017/s003329172100146x.
22 Hayley Young, Jason Davies, and David Benton, "Non-Suicidal Self-Injury Is Associated with Multidimensional Deficits in Interoception: Evidence from Three Studies," preprint, PsyArXiv, April 24, 2019, 28, https://doi.org/10.31234/osf.io/2azer.
23 Lisa M. Störkel, Alexander Karabatsiakis, Johanna Hepp, Iris-Tatjana Kolassa, Christian Schmahl, and Inga Niedtfeld, "Salivary Beta-Endorphin in Nonsuicidal Self-Injury: An Ambulatory Assessment Study," *Neuropsychopharmacology* 46 (January 2021): 1361, https://doi.org/10.1038/s41386-020-00914-2.
24 M. Shae Nester, Nicholas A. Pierorazio, Gavi Shandler, and Bethany L. Brand, "Characteristics, Methods, and Functions of Non-Suicidal Self-Injury Among Highly Dissociative Individuals," *Journal of Trauma and Dissociation* 24, no. 3 (2023): 333, https://doi.org/10.1080/15299732.2023.2181475.
25 Lorenzo Lucherini Angeletti, Emanuele Cassioli, Livio Tarchi, Cristiano Dani, Marco Faldi, Rachele Martini, et al., "From Early Relational Experiences to Non-Suicidal Self-Injury in Anorexia and Bulimia Nervosa: A Structural Equation Model Unraveling the Role of Impairments in Interoception," *Eating and Weight Disorders* 29, no. 22 (2024): 3, https://doi.org/10.1007/s40519-024-01651-x.
26 Nester et al., "Characteristics, Methods, and Functions," 344.
27 Young et al., "Non-Suicidal Self-Injury," 26.

## Chapter 15: Substance Use and Addiction Disorders

1 Substance Abuse and Mental Health Services Administration, *Key Substance Use and Mental Health Indicators in the United States: Results from the 2024 National Survey on Drug Use and Health* (Center for Behavioral Health Statistics and Quality, 2025), 24, www.samhsa.gov/data/sites/default/files/reports/rpt56287/2024-nsduh-annual-national-report.pdf.
2 Zainab Alimoradi, Aida Lotfi, Chung-Ying Lin, Mark D. Griffiths, and Amir H. Pakpour, "Estimation of Behavioral Addiction Prevalence During COVID-19 Pandemic: A Systematic Review and Meta-Analysis," *Current Addiction Reports* 9 (September 2022): 486, https://doi.org/10.1007/s40429-022-00435-6.
3 Gabor Maté, *In the Realm of Hungry Ghosts: Close Encounters with Addiction* (North Atlantic Books, 2010), 33.
4 Vincent J. Felitti, Robert F. Anda, Dale Nordenberg, Valerie Edwards, Mary P. Koss, James S. Marks, et al., "Relationship of Childhood Abuse and Household Dysfunction to Many of the Leading Causes of Death in Adults: The Adverse Childhood Experiences (ACE) Study," *American Journal of Preventive Medicine* 14, no. 4 (1998): 245, https://doi.org/10.1016/s0749-3797(98)00017-8.
5 Barna Konkolÿ Thege, David C. Hodgins, and T. Cameron Wild, "Co-Occurring Substance-Related and Behavioral Addiction Problems: A Person-Centered, Lay Epidemiology Approach," *Journal of Behavioral Addictions* 5, no. 4 (2016): 619, https://doi.org/10.1556/2006.5.2016.079.

6 Eszter Kotyuk, Anna Magi, Andrea Eisinger, Orsolya Király, Andrea Vereczkei, Csaba Barta, et al., "Co-Occurrences of Substance Use and Other Potentially Addictive Behaviors: Epidemiological Results from the Psychological and Genetic Factors of the Addictive Behaviors (PGA) Study," *Journal of Behavioral Addictions* 9, no. 2 (2020): 272, https://doi.org/10.1556/2006.2020.00033.
7 Pauline Billaux, Shailendra Segobin, Angeline Maillard, Vanessa Bloch, Christine Delmaire, Nicolas Cabé, Alice Laniepce, et al., "Let's Focus on the Insula in Addiction: A Refined Anatomical Exploration of Insula in Severe Alcohol and Cocaine Use Disorders," *European Psychiatry* 67, no. 1 (2024): e75, https://doi.org/10.1192/j.eurpsy.2024.1784.
8 Aleksandra M. Herman and Theodora Duka, "Facets of Impulsivity and Alcohol Use: What Role Do Emotions Play?," *Neuroscience and Biobehavioral Reviews* 106 (November 2019): 202–16, https://doi.org/10.1016/j.neubiorev.2018.08.011.
9 Francesco Di Carlo, Maria Chiara Vicinelli, Mauro Pettorruso, Luisa De Risio, Giuseppe Migliara, Valentina Baccolini, et al., "Connected Minds in Disconnected Bodies: Exploring the Role of Interoceptive Sensibility and Alexithymia in Problematic Use of the Internet," *Comprehensive Psychiatry* 129 (February 2024): 152446, https://doi.org/10.1016/j.comppsych.2023.152446.
10 Francesca Gioia, Valeria Rega, and Valentina Boursier, "Problematic Internet Use and Emotional Dysregulation Among Young People: A Literature Review," *Clinical Neuropsychiatry* 18, no. 1 (2021): 47, https://doi.org/10.36131/cnfioritieditore20210104.
11 Georgia Panayiotou, Tonia-Flery Artemi, Marios Theodorou, Christiana Theodorou, and Klavdia Neophytou, "Not 'Just for Fun': Gambling, Substance Use, and the Transdiagnostic Role of Emotion Regulation," *Cogent Psychology* 10, no. 1 (2023), https://doi.org/10.1080/23311908.2023.2183677.
12 Aleksandra M. Herman, "Interoception Within the Context of Impulsivity and Addiction," *Current Addiction Reports* 10 (April 2023): 97–106, https://doi.org/10.1007/s40429-023-00482-7.
13 Herman, "Interoception."
14 Herman and Duka, "Facets of Impulsivity and Alcohol Use."
15 Daniela Marchetti, Maria Cristina Verrocchio, and Piero Porcelli, "Gambling Problems and Alexithymia: A Systematic Review," *Brain Sciences* 9, no. 8 (2019): 191, https://doi.org/10.3390/brainsci9080191.
16 Di Carlo et al., "Connected Minds in Disconnected Bodies."
17 Lieke M. J. Swinkels, Harm Veling, and Hein T. van Schie, "Playing Videogames Is Associated with Reduced Awareness of Bodily Sensations," *Computers in Human Behavior* 125 (December 2021): 106953, https://doi.org/10.1016/j.chb.2021.106953.
18 Işıl Ateş Çöl, Mehmet Bülent Sönmez, and Mehmet Erdal Vardar, "Evaluation of Interoceptive Awareness in Alcohol-Addicted Patients," *Archives of Neuropsychiatry* 53, no. 1 (2016): 18, https://pmc.ncbi.nlm.nih.gov/articles/PMC5353231.
19 Martin P. Paulus and Jennifer L. Stewart, "Interoception and Drug Addiction," *Neuropharmacology* 76 (January 2014): 342–50, https://doi.org/10.1016/j.neuropharm.2013.07.002.
20 Herman, "Interoception," 101.
21 Shikha Shukla and Cynthia L. Hsu, "Alcohol Use Disorder and the Gut–Brain Axis: A Narrative Review of the Role of Gut Microbiota and Implications for Treatment," *Microorganisms* 13, no. 1 (2025): 67, https://doi.org/10.3390/microorganisms13010067.
22 Herman, "Interoception."

## Chapter 16: Disordered Eating


1 Phillipa Hay, Phillip Aouad, Anvi Le, Peta Marks, Danielle Maloney, National Eating Disorder Research Consortium, et al., "Epidemiology of Eating Disorders: Population, Prevalence, Disease Burden, and Quality of Life Informing Public Policy in Australia—A Rapid Review," *Journal of Eating Disorders* 11, no. 23 (2023), https://doi.org/10.1186/s40337-023-00738-7.

2 José Francisco López-Gil, Antonio García-Hermoso, Lee Smith, Joseph Firth, Mike Trott, Arthur Eumann Mesas, et al., "Global Proportion of Disordered Eating in Children and Adolescents: A Systematic Review and Meta-Analysis," *JAMA Pediatrics* 177, no. 4 (2023): 363, https://doi.org/10.1001/jamapediatrics.2022.5848.

3 Alexandra D. Convertino and Rebecca R. Mendoza, "Posttraumatic Stress Disorder, Traumatic Events, and Longitudinal Eating Disorder Treatment Outcomes: A Systematic Review," *International Journal of Eating Disorders* 56, no. 6 (2023): 1056, https://doi.org/10.1002/eat.23933.

4 Irina A. Vanzhula, Benjamin Calebs, Laura Fewell, and Cheri A. Levinson, "Illness Pathways Between Eating Disorder and Post-Traumatic Stress Disorder Symptoms: Understanding Comorbidity with Network Analysis," *European Eating Disorders Review* 27, no. 2 (2018): 148, https://doi.org/10.1002/erv.2634.

5 Convertino and Mendoza, "Posttraumatic Stress Disorder," 1056.

6 Convertino and Mendoza, "Posttraumatic Stress Disorder," 1057.

7 Lorenzo Lucherini Angeletti, Emanuele Cassioli, Livio Tarchi, Cristiano Dani, Marco Faldi, Rachele Martini, et al., "From Early Relational Experiences to Non-Suicidal Self-Injury in Anorexia and Bulimia Nervosa: A Structural Equation Model Unraveling the Role of Impairments in Interoception," *Eating and Weight Disorders* 29, no. 22 (2024), https://doi.org/10.1007/s40519-024-01651-x.

8 Alessio Maria Monteleone, Giammarco Cascino, Matteo Martini, Giuseppina Patriciello, Valeria Ruzzi, Nadia Delsedime, et al., "Confidence in One-Self and Confidence in One's Own Body: The Revival of an Old Paradigm for Anorexia Nervosa," *Clinical Psychology and Psychotherapy* 28, no. 4 (2020): 823, https://doi.org/10.1002/cpp.2535.

9 Monteleone et al., "Confidence in One-Self."

10 Jenni Leppanen, Dalia Brown, Hannah McLinden, Steven Williams, and Kate Tchanturia, "The Role of Emotion Regulation in Eating Disorders: A Network Meta-Analysis Approach," *Frontiers in Psychiatry* 13 (February 2022): 793094, https://doi.org/10.3389/fpsyt.2022.793094.

11 Leppanen et al., "Role of Emotion Regulation."

12 Aline Tiemann, Marius Rubo, Sarah N. Garfinkel, Claus Vögele, Zoé van Dyck, and Simone Munsch, "Listening to Your Stomach: Effects of Gastric Biofeedback Training on Interoception, Eating Behavior and Eating Disorder Symptoms," *Physiology and Behavior* 302 (December 2025): 115108, https://doi.org/10.1016/j.physbeh.2025.115108.

13 Carina Carlucci Palazzo, Barbara Esteves Leghi, and Rosa Wanda Diez-Garcia, "Food Consciousness Intervention Improves Interoceptive Sensitivity and Expression of Exteroception in Women," *Nutrients* 14, no. 3 (January 2022): 450, https://doi.org/10.3390/nu14030450.

14 Palazzo et al., "Food Consciousness Intervention."

15 Giulia Brizzi, Maria Sansoni, Daniele Di Lernia, Fabio Frisone, Cosimo Tuena, and Giuseppe Riva, "The Multisensory Mind: A Systematic Review of Multisensory Integration Processing in Anorexia and Bulimia Nervosa," *Journal of Eating Disorders* 11, no. 204 (2023), https://doi.org/10.1186/s40337-023-00930-9.

16 Laura Case, "A GI-Interoceptive Threat Theory of Restrictive Eating: Insights from Active Inference and Chronic Pain," *Brain and Behavior* 15, no. 9 (2025): e70892, https://doi.org/10.1002/brb3.70892.
17 Monteleone et al., "Confidence in One-Self," 824.
18 Janell L. Mensinger, Arjena Valls Palacios Reese, Alexandria Johnston, and Katerina Rinaldi, "Eating Pathology and Interoceptive Sensibility Using the Brief Multidimensional Assessment of Interoceptive Awareness-2: Can There Be Too Much of a Good Thing?," *Journal of Personality Assessment* 107, no. 5 (2025): 671–83. https://doi.org/10.1080/00223891.2024.2445706.

## Chapter 17: Neurodivergent Conditions

1 Kelly Mahler, *Interoception: The Eighth Sensory System* (AAPC Publishing, 2015).
2 Saray Bonete, Clara Molinero, and Daniela Ruisanchez, "Emotional Dysfunction and Interoceptive Challenges in Adults with Autism Spectrum Disorders," *Behavioral Sciences* 13, no. 4 (2023): 312, https://doi.org/10.3390/bs13040312.
3 Marlene Klein, Michael Witthöft, and Stefanie Maria Jungmann, "Interoception in Individuals with Autism Spectrum Disorder: A Systematic Literature Review and Meta-Analysis," *Frontiers in Psychiatry* 16 (August 2025): 1573263, https://doi.org/10.3389/fpsyt.2025.1573263.
4 Chihiro Itoi, Yuta Ujiie, Yuuki Ooishi, and Makio Kashino, "The Relationship Between Subjective Difficulty in Interoceptive Processing and Accuracy of Heartbeat Perception in Autistic Individuals," *Discover Mental Health* 4, no. 13 (2024), https://doi.org/10.1007/s44192-024-00065-6.
5 Kelly Mahler, Kerri Hample, Claudia Jones, Joseph Sensenig, Phoebe Thomasco, and Claudia Hilton, "Impact of an Interoception-Based Program on Emotion Regulation in Autistic Children," *Occupational Therapy International*, April 20, 2022, https://doi.org/10.1155/2022/9328967.
6 Nour Ben Hassen, Francisco Molins, Dolores Garrote-Petisco, and Miguel Ángel Serrano, "Emotional Regulation Deficits in Autism Spectrum Disorder: The Role of Alexithymia and Interoception," *Research in Developmental Disabilities* 132 (January 2023): 104378, https://doi.org/10.1016/j.ridd.2022.104378.
7 Jessie Poquérusse, Luigi Pastore, Sara Dellantonio, and Gianluca Esposito, "Alexithymia and Autism Spectrum Disorder: A Complex Relationship," *Frontiers in Psychology* 9 (July 2018): 1196, https://doi.org/10.3389/fpsyg.2018.01196.
8 Bruna Santos da Silva, Eugenio Horacio Grevet, Luiza Carolina Fagundes Silva, João Kleber Neves Ramos, Diego Luiz Rovaris, and Claiton Henrique Dotto Bau, "An Overview on Neurobiology and Therapeutics of Attention-Deficit/Hyperactivity Disorder," *Discover Mental Health* 3, no. 2 (2023), https://doi.org/10.1007/s44192-022-00030-1.
9 Artemios Pehlivanidis, Katerina Papanikolaou, Vasilios Mantas, Eva Kalantzi, Kalliopi Korobili, Lida-Alkisti Xenaki, et al., "Lifetime Co-Occurring Psychiatric Disorders in Newly Diagnosed Adults with Attention Deficit Hyperactivity Disorder (ADHD) or/and Autism Spectrum Disorder (ASD)," *BMC Psychiatry* 20, 423 (2020), https://doi.org/10.1186/s12888-020-02828-1.
10 Santos da Silva et al., "Overview on Neurobiology."
11 Santos da Silva et al., "Overview on Neurobiology."
12 Valeria Isaac, Vladimir Lopez, and Maria Josefina Escobar, "Arousal Dysregulation and Executive Dysfunction in Attention Deficit Hyperactivity Disorder (ADHD),"

*Frontiers in Psychiatry* 14 (January 2024): 1336040, https://doi.org/10.3389/fpsyt.2023.1336040.

13 Isaac et al., "Arousal Dysregulation"; Ceren Turkoglu, Feyza Okyaz, and Elif Arslan, "The Relationship Between ADHD and Autonomic Regulation: A Pupillometry-Based Study," *Bratislava Medical Journal* 126 (May 2025): 1962, https://doi.org/10.1007/s44411-025-00185-7.

14 Nicole M. Brown, Suzette N. Brown, Rahil D. Briggs, Miguelina Germán, Peter F. Belamarich, and Suzette O. Oyeku, "Associations Between Adverse Childhood Experiences and ADHD Diagnosis and Severity," *Academic Pediatrics* 17, no. 4 (2017): 353, https://doi.org/10.1016/j.acap.2016.08.013.

15 Magda Wojtara, Yusra Syeda, Heshwin Singh, Emaan Rana, and Saleem Sabeer, "Examining Adverse Childhood Experiences and Attention Deficit/Hyperactivity Disorder: A Systematic Review," *Mental Health Science* 1, no. 2 (2023): 110, https://doi.org/10.1002/mhs2.26.

16 Ana-María Soler-Gutiérrez, Juan-Carlos Pérez-González, and Julia Mayas, "Evidence of Emotion Dysregulation as a Core Symptom of Adult ADHD: A Systematic Review," *PLOS ONE* 18, no. 1 (2023): e0280131, https://doi.org/10.1371/journal.pone.0280131.

17 Begum Yulug Tas, Gonca Ozyurt, Oyku Yavuz Kan, and Gozde Ulas, "The Sensory Dimension of Attention Deficit Hyperactivity Disorder: A Case–Control Study on the Impact of Sensory Profile on Daily Functioning Among Turkish Children with ADHD," *Middle East Current Psychiatry* 32, no. 76 (2025), https://doi.org/10.1186/s43045-025-00569-z.

18 Yulug Tas et al., "Sensory Dimension."

19 Lía Martínez, Edward Prada, Corina Satler, Maria C. H. Tavares, and Carlos Tomaz, "Executive Dysfunctions: The Role in Attention Deficit Hyperactivity and Post-Traumatic Stress Neuropsychiatric Disorders," *Frontiers in Psychology* 7 (August 2016): 1230, https://doi.org/10.3389/fpsyg.2016.01230.

20 Ümit Başar Semiz, Özgür Öner , Fatma Fariha Cengiz, and Mustafa Bilici, "Childhood Abuse and Neglect in Adult Attention-Deficit/Hyperactivity Disorder," *Psychiatry and Clinical Psychopharmacology* 27, no. 4 (2017): 344, https://doi.org/10.1080/24750573.2017.1367551.

21 Brown et al., "Associations Between Adverse Childhood Experiences," 353.

22 Anna Grossman and Avi Avital, "Emotional and Sensory Dysregulation as a Possible Missing Link in Attention Deficit Hyperactivity Disorder: A Review," *Frontiers in Behavioral Neuroscience* 17 (March 2023): 1118937, https://doi.org/10.3389/fnbeh.2023.1118937.

23 Wojtara et al., "Examining Adverse Childhood Experiences," 110.

24 Linlin Fan and Tinghu Kang, "Early Childhood Trauma and Its Long-Term Impact on Cognitive and Emotional Development: A Systematic Review and Meta-Analysis," *Annals of Medicine* 57, no. 1 (2025), https://doi.org/10.1080/07853890.2025.2536199.

## Chapter 18: Physical Health

1 Camilla L. Nord and Sarah N. Garfinkel, "Interoceptive Pathways to Understand and Treat Mental Health Conditions," *Trends in Cognitive Sciences* 26, no. 6 (2022): 504, https://doi.org/10.1016/j.tics.2022.03.004.

2 Nord and Garfinkel, "Interoceptive Pathways," 504.

3 Vincent J. Felitti, Robert F. Anda, Dale Nordenberg, Valerie Edwards, Mary P. Koss, James S. Marks, et al., "Relationship of Childhood Abuse and Household Dysfunction to Many of the Leading Causes of Death in Adults: The Adverse Childhood Experiences (ACE) Study," *American Journal of Preventive Medicine* 14, no. 4 (1998): 245, https://doi.org/10.1016/s0749-3797(98)00017-8.
4 Dana Dharmakaya Colgan, Ashley Eddy, Kaylie Green, and Barry Oken, "Adaptive Body Awareness Predicts Fewer Central Sensitization–Related Symptoms and Explains Relationship Between Central Sensitization–Related Symptoms and Pain Intensity: A Cross-Sectional Study Among Individuals with Chronic Pain," *Pain Practice* 22, no. 2 (2022): 223, https://doi.org/10.1111/papr.13083.
5 Colgan et al., "Adaptive Body Awareness," 225.
6 Zuhal Koc Apaydin, "Somatosensory Amplification: Conceptual Structure, Neurobiological Foundations, and Clinical Implications," *Journal of Clinical and Basic Psychosomatics*, August 8, 2025, https://doi.org/10.36922/jcbp025260047.
7 Annabel Horsburgh, Simon J. Summers, Aidan Lewis, Richard J. Keegan, and Andrew Flood, "The Relationship Between Pain and Interoception: A Systematic Review and Meta-Analysis," *Journal of Pain* 25, no. 7 (2024): 104476, https://doi.org/10.1016/j.jpain.2024.01.341.
8 Alexander M. Dydyk, Emmanuel Chiebuka, Michael F. Stretanski, and Amy Givler, *Central Pain Syndrome* (StatPearls Publishing, 2025), www.ncbi.nlm.nih.gov/books/NBK553027.
9 Colgan et al., "Adaptive Body Awareness," 223.
10 Dydyk et al., *Central Pain Syndrome.*
11 Colgan et al., "Adaptive Body Awareness," 223.
12 Giuseppe Marano, Gianandrea Traversi, Roberto Pola, Antonio Gasbarrini, Eleonora Gaetani, and Marianna Mazza, "Irritable Bowel Syndrome: A Hallmark of Psychological Distress in Women?," *Life* 15, no. 2 (2025): 277, https://doi.org/10.3390/life15020277.
13 Katerina Karaivazoglou, Ioanna Aggeletopoulou, and Christos Triantos, "Interoceptive Processing in Functional Gastrointestinal Disorders," *International Journal of Molecular Sciences* 25, no. 14 (2024): 7633, https://doi.org/10.3390/ijms25147633.
14 Alicia Fournier, Laurie Mondillon, Olivier Luminet, Fréderic Canini, Nicolas Mathieu, Anne Sophie Gauchez, et al., "Interoceptive Abilities in Inflammatory Bowel Diseases and Irritable Bowel Syndrome," *Frontiers in Psychiatry* 11 (April 2020): 229, https://doi.org/10.3389/fpsyt.2020.00229.
15 Karaivazoglou et al., "Interoceptive Processing."
16 Ewa Dudzińska, Andreas M. Grabrucker, Paweł Kwiatkowski, Robert Sitarz, and Monika Sienkiewicz, "The Importance of Visceral Hypersensitivity in Irritable Bowel Syndrome—Plant Metabolites in IBS Treatment," *Pharmaceuticals* 16, no. 10 (2023): 1405, https://doi.org/10.3390/ph16101405.
17 Jacek Kolacz and Stephen W. Porges, "Chronic Diffuse Pain and Functional Gastrointestinal Disorders After Traumatic Stress: Pathophysiology Through a Polyvagal Perspective," *Frontiers in Medicine* 5 (May 2018): 145, https://doi.org/10.3389/fmed.2018.00145.
18 Dudzińska et al., "Importance of Visceral Hypersensitivity."
19 Fournier et al., "Interoceptive Abilities."
20 Marano et al., "Irritable Bowel Syndrome."
21 Kolacz and Porges, "Chronic Diffuse Pain."

22 Marano et al., "Irritable Bowel Syndrome."
23 Marano et al., "Irritable Bowel Syndrome."
24 Sabrina Berens, Rainer Schaefert, Johannes C. Ehrenthal, David Baumeister, Wolfgang Eich, and Jonas Tesarz, "Different Dimensions of Affective Processing in Patients with Irritable Bowel Syndrome: A Multi-Center Cross-Sectional Study," *Frontiers in Psychology* 12 (March 2021): 625381, https://doi.org/10.3389/fpsyg.2021.625381.
25 Keisuke Suzuki, Shiho Suzuki, Tomohiko Shiina, Madoka Okamura, Yasuo Haruyama, Muneto Tatsumoto, et al., "Investigating the Relationships Between the Burden of Multiple Sensory Hypersensitivity Symptoms and Headache-Related Disability in Patients with Migraine," *Journal of Headache and Pain* 22, no. 77 (2021), https://doi.org/10.1186/s10194-021-01294-8.
26 Suzuki et al., "Investigating the Relationships."
27 Suzuki et al., "Investigating the Relationships."
28 Akihiro Koreki, Vilomi Bhatia, Anne-Marie Logan, Usman Khan, Mitsumoto Onaya, Sarah Garfinkel, et al., "Interoception and Dissociation in Migraine: A Case–Control Study of Chronic and Episodic Subtypes," *Frontiers in Neurology* 16 (August 2025): 1643260, https://doi.org/10.3389/fneur.2025.1643260.
29 Koreki et al., "Interoception and Dissociation in Migraine."
30 Koreki et al., "Interoception and Dissociation in Migraine."

## Chapter 19: Interpersonal Connections

1 Deb Dana, *The Polyvagal Theory in Therapy: Engaging the Rhythm of Regulation* (Norton, 2018), 46.
2 Kristina Oldroyd, Monisha Pasupathi, and Cecilia Wainryb, "Social Antecedents to the Development of Interoception: Attachment Related Processes Are Associated with Interoception," *Frontiers in Psychology* 10 (April 2019): 712, https://doi.org/10.3389/fpsyg.2019.00712.
3 Oldroyd et al., "Social Antecedents."
4 Clare E. Palmer and Manos Tsakiris, "Going at the Heart of Social Cognition: Is There a Role for Interoception in Self-Other Distinction?," *Current Opinion in Psychology* 24 (December 2018): 21–26, https://doi.org/10.1016/j.copsyc.2018.04.008.
5 Mallory J. Feldman, Ruofan Ma, and Kristen A. Lindquist, "The Role of Interoception in Emotion and Social Cognition," in *Interoception*, ed. Jennifer Murphy and Rebecca Brewer (Springer, 2024), 125–49, https://doi.org/10.1007/978-3-031-68521-7_5.
6 Felix Schoeller, Leonardo Christov-Moore, and Nicco Reggente, "Emotional Contagion: The Role of Interoceptive Inference in Affective Empathy and Co-Regulation," preprint, PsyArXiv, December 9, 2024, 7, https://doi.org/10.31234/osf.io/6gf59.
7 Larissa Medeiros Leão, Amalia Cinthia Meneses Rêgo, and Irami Araújo-Filho, "Interoception: Current Knowledge Gaps and Future Directions in Neuroscience, Psychopathology, and Clinical Applications," *International Journal of Innovative Research in Medical Science* 10, no. 3 (2025): 108, https://doi.org/10.23958/ijirms/vol10-i03/2041.
8 Feldman et al., "Role of Interoception," 137.
9 Delphine Grynberg and Olga Pollatos, "Perceiving One's Body Shapes Empathy," *Physiology and Behavior* 140 (March 2015): 58, https://doi.org/10.1016/j.physbeh.2014.12.026.
10 Wendy D'Andrea, Nadia Nieves, and Treva Van Cleave, "To Thine Own Self Be True: Interoceptive Accuracy and Interpersonal Problems," *Borderline Personality Disorder*

*and Emotion Dysregulation* 9, no. 6 (2022), https://doi.org/10.1186/s40479-021-00175-5.

11 Schoeller et al., "Emotional Contagion," 7.

12 Jeffrey A. Bouffard and Holly A. Miller, "The Role of Sexual Arousal and Overperception of Sexual Intent Within the Decision to Engage in Sexual Coercion," *Journal of Interpersonal Violence* 29, no. 11 (2014): 1967–86, https://doi.org/10.1177/0886260513515950.

13 Allan N. Schore, *Affect Regulation and the Origin of the Self: The Neurobiology of Emotional Development* (Routledge, 2015).

14 Antonio Damasio, *Descartes' Error: Emotion, Reason, and the Human Brain* (Penguin Books, 2005).

15 Gallup and Meta, *The Global State of Social Connections* (Gallup, 2023), www.gallup.com/analytics/509675/state-of-social-connections.aspx, 2.

16 Lisa Quadt, Giulia Esposito, Hugo D. Critchley, and Sarah N. Garfinkel, "Brain-Body Interactions Underlying the Association of Loneliness with Mental and Physical Health," *Neuroscience and Biobehavioral Reviews* 116 (September 2020): 283–300, https://doi.org/10.1016/j.neubiorev.2020.06.015.

17 Quadt et al., "Brain-Body Interactions."

18 Quadt et al., "Brain-Body Interactions."

## Chapter 20: Determining What's Helpful

1 *"Multidimensional Assessment of Interoceptive Awareness,"* University of California San Francisco Osher Center for Integrative Health, accessed January 4, 2026, https://osher.ucsf.edu/research/maia.

## Chapter 22: Practitioner-Led Therapies and Approaches

1 Adam W. Hanley, Wolf E. Mehling, and Eric L. Garland, "Holding the Body in Mind: Interoceptive Awareness, Dispositional Mindfulness and Psychological Well-Being," *Journal of Psychosomatic Research* 99 (August 2017): 13, https://doi.org/10.1016/j.jpsychores.2017.05.014.

2 Jonathan Gibson, "Mindfulness, Interoception, and the Body: A Contemporary Perspective," *Frontiers in Psychology* 10 (September 2019): 2012, https://doi.org/10.3389/fpsyg.2019.02012.

3 Sylwia Sumińska and Andrzej Rynkiewicz, "Mindfulness-Based Stress Reduction Training Supplemented with Physiological Signals from Smartwatch Improves Mindfulness and Reduces Stress, but Not Anxiety and Depression," *PLOS ONE* 20, no. 4 (2025): e0322413, https://doi.org/10.1371/journal.pone.0322413.

4 Evgenia Gkintoni, Stephanos P. Vassilopoulos, and Georgios Nikolaou, "Mindfulness-Based Cognitive Therapy in Clinical Practice: A Systematic Review of Neurocognitive Outcomes and Applications for Mental Health and Well-Being," *Journal of Clinical Medicine* 14, no. 5 (2025): 1703, https://doi.org/10.3390/jcm14051703.

5 Steven C. Hayes, Jacqueline Pistorello, and Michael E. Levin, "Acceptance and Commitment Therapy as a Unified Model of Behavior Change," *The Counseling Psychologist* 40, no. 7 (2012): 976–1002, https://doi.org/10.1177/0011000012460836.

6 Peter A. Levine, *Waking the Tiger: Healing Trauma* (North Atlantic Books, 1997).

7 "About," Sensorimotor Psychotherapy Institute, accessed January 5, 2026, https://sensorimotorpsychotherapy.org/about.

8 Caitlin Anna Laycox, "An Empirical Framework for Interoceptive Sensibility as a Transdiagnostic Feature of Autonomic Regulation: A Potential Mediator of Trauma-Related Psychopathology and Somatic Mindfulness Intervention Effects" (PhD diss., Southern Cross University, 2024), 25, https://doi.org/10.25918/thesis.534.

9 David Emerson, Kristen Pringle, Maria Jude, Evan Bodine, Edwina Kempe, and Viann N. Nguyen-Feng, "Trauma Center Trauma-Sensitive Yoga: Conceptual Components, Facilitation Guides, and Reflections," in *The Palgrave Handbook of Third-Wave Psychotherapies*, ed. Wendy Wen Li, Gemma M. Griffith, Shauna Shapiro, and Zhuohong Zhu (Palgrave Macmillan, 2025), 826, https://doi.org/10.1007/978-3-032-00353-9_34.

10 Emerson et al., "Trauma Center Trauma-Sensitive Yoga."

11 "What Is DBT?," *Behavioral Tech Institute,* accessed January 5, 2026, https://behavioraltech.org/dialectical-behavior-therapy-dbt.

12 Samantha G. Farris, Lilly Derby, and Mindy M. Kibbey, "Getting Comfortable with Physical Discomfort: A Scoping Review of Interoceptive Exposure in Physical and Mental Health Conditions," *Psychological Bulletin* 151, no. 2 (2025): 131–33, https://doi.org/10.1037/bul0000464.

13 Farris et al., "Getting Comfortable," 131–33.

14 Farris et al., "Getting Comfortable," 131–33.

15 Farris et al., "Getting Comfortable," 173.

# Index


## A

acceptance and commitment therapy (ACT), 7, 231, 233–234
addiction. *See* substance use and addiction disorders
ADHD (attention deficit hyperactivity disorder), 51–52, 169, 172–177
Adverse Childhood Experiences (ACE) Study, 8, 86, 113–114, 152–153, 175, 180
agency, 27
Ainsworth, Mary, 68
alcohol use disorder. *See* substance use and addiction disorders
Alexander, F. M., 7
alexithymia, 101–102, 156, 172
amygdala, 76, 83, 130
analytic paralysis, 32
anorexia nervosa, 145, 162–164, 166. *See also* disordered eating
anterior insular cortex (AIC), 16
anxiety disorders
- depression and, 134
- increase in, 119
- interoception and, 120–125
- MAIA domains impacted by, 126–127
- prediction errors and, 125–126
- prevalence of, 120
- types of, 119

anxious depression, 132–136, 138
asthma, 28, 53
attachment
- brain development and, 71
- co-regulation and, 67–68
- definition of, 67
- emotional regulation and, 196
- interoception and, 69–70, 74, 192

attachment styles
- in adulthood, 72–74
- anxious, 69, 71, 72–73
- avoidant, 69, 71, 73–74
- development of, 68–69
- insecure, 69, 70–74, 112–113, 162–163
- interoception shaped by, 70–71
- secure, 69, 70

attachment theory, history of, 68
attention regulation (MAIA domain)
- ADHD and, 176–177
- autism and, 176
- interpreting scores for, 210
- overview of, with examples, 41–42
- trauma and, 100–101

autism spectrum disorder (ASD), 52, 169–172, 176–177
autoimmune disorders, 52–53, 78, 179
autonomic nervous system (ANS), 17–19, 75–76
autonomic regulation, 17–19
avoidance
- anxiety disorders and, 123–126
- chronic stress and, 83
- as coping behavior, 117
- depression and, 135–136
- trauma and, 91, 94

## B

Barrett, Lisa Feldman, 62
binge eating, 162. *See also* disordered eating

body awareness, maladaptive, 181–182
body dysmorphic disorder (BDD), 141, 144–146
body listening (MAIA domain)
  disordered eating and, 167
  interpreting scores for, 211–212
  overview of, with examples, 44–45
  trauma and, 103–104
body scan, 222–223
body sensations
  excessive worry about, 61–62
  hyperattention to, 121–122, 135
  labeling, 218–219
  language of, 219–222
  misinterpreting, 58–59, 122–123, 135
  noticing comfortable and neutral, 223
body tracking practices, 215–223
Bowlby, John, 68
brain. *See also individual parts*
  connection of gut and, 16, 53–55, 131, 184–185
  development of, and attachment, 71
  as forecaster, 20–22
  interoception and, 19–20
breath tracking practices, 223–224
bulimia, 162, 164. *See also* disordered eating
busyness, 83
butterfly tapping, 226

## C

Cameron, William Bruce, 37
cardiovascular disease, 53, 111, 130, 179, 233
cardiovascular system
  chronic stress and, 78
  depression and, 130
  interoceptive signals from, 13
case studies
  Ava (aspiring fashion influencer), 9–10, 33, 39–46, 59, 62, 74, 88–92, 113, 146, 148, 158, 163
  Catherine (nurse with high standards), 9, 30, 33, 39–46, 59–61, 64–65, 82, 89–91, 94, 116, 124, 159
  David (depressed business owner), 10, 39–41, 43–44, 59–62, 82, 93–95, 137, 159, 198
  Hailey (struggling with health anxiety), 10, 39–46, 50–51, 59–60, 62, 64, 72–73, 82, 122, 133, 188
  Jason (construction worker with quick temper), 10, 31–32, 39–46, 50, 59–60, 64, 89–90, 92, 94, 114, 146, 159
  Lauren (committed preschool teacher), 10, 32, 34, 39–46, 50–51, 59–61, 72, 82, 164, 186, 195
  Roland (accountant with failing marriage), 9, 30–31, 39–42, 44–45, 50–51, 59–60, 64, 74, 81–82, 93–94, 102, 117
Centers for Disease Control (CDC), 57
central sensitization (CS), 182
chronic fatigue syndrome, 28, 78, 100, 182
chronic stress
  behaviors resulting from, 83–84
  definition of, 80
  examples of, 81–82
  gut microbes and, 54
  interoceptive disruptions and, 8, 79–80
  physical effects of, 75, 77–78
cognitive behavioral therapy (CBT), 7, 57
cognitive defusion, 233, 234
cognitive distortions, 57–58, 64–65
contamination OCD, 144
COPD (chronic obstructive pulmonary disease), 53, 75
coping behaviors, 91–92, 115–117, 153–154, 157–160
co-regulation, 67–68, 192–193
cortisol, 76–78, 80, 120, 184, 232
COVID, 52, 179
Craig, Bud, 16, 25, 28
cravings, 156

## D


Damasio, Antonio, 25
decision-making, 24–25, 31–32
default mode network (DMN), 101
depression
anxious, 132–133, 132–136, 138
body's role in, 130–131
comorbidity and, 134
fatigue and, 131–132
interoception and, 134–138
MAIA domains impacted by, 138–139
motivation and, 137–138
nervous system and, 130, 133–134
prevalence of, 129
symptoms of, 129
Descartes, René, 25
Desmedt, Olivier, 37
diabetes, 52–53, 55, 75, 78, 111, 116, 134, 179
dialectical behavior therapy (DBT), 238–239
disgust proneness, 144
disordered eating
anxiety and, 124–125
as coping tool, 115–116
eating disorders vs., 161
impact of external cues on, 164–166
insecure attachment and, 162–163
interoceptive challenges in, 163–166
MAIA domains impacted by, 166–167
prevalence of, 161
spectrum of, 162
trauma and, 162–163
dissociation, 18, 92–93, 104, 148, 175–176, 200, 231, 234–236, 239
distraction. *See also* not-distracting (MAIA domain)
addiction and, 116
anxiety disorders and, 123–124
depression and, 135–136
drug use. *See* substance use and addiction disorders
Dunne, Julie, 137
dysbiosis, 54, 131


## E


eating disorders, 161. *See also* disordered eating
Eggart, Michael, 131
egomania, 33
embodied cognition, 26, 193
embodied emotions, 24
EMDR (eye movement desensitization and reprocessing), 234, 235–236
emotional awareness (MAIA domain)
ADHD and, 177
autism and, 177
depression and, 138–139
interoception and, 24
interpersonal connections and, 199
interpreting scores for, 211
overview of, with examples, 42–43
trauma and, 101–102
emotional differentiation, 24
emotional reactivity, 84
emotional regulation
addiction and, 155
attachment and, 196
autism and, 171–172
disordered eating and, 163–164
interoception and, 24
emotions
affective interoceptive messages and, 5
alexithymia, 101–102, 156, 172
dampened, 93
disconnection from, 31
embodied, 24
insula and, 16
intensity of, 24, 31
interoception and, 23–24, 30–31
suppressing, 60, 83, 117
thinking and, 25, 60
trauma and, 89–90, 93

empathy, 34, 193–196
endocrine system
  chronic stress and, 78
  interoceptive signals from, 14
enmeshment, 195
exaggerating, patterns of, 59–60
excoriation disorder. *See* skin-picking disorder

## F

Farris, Samantha, 240
Feldenkrais, Moshé, 7
Felitti, Vincent, 86
felt sense, 219
fibromyalgia, 51, 78, 99, 100, 180, 182
fight-or-flight response, 18, 76–77, 81, 89
flashbacks, 81, 87, 90, 235
fullness cues, 164

## G

Ganci, Michael, 54
Garfinkel, Sarah, 37
gastrointestinal system
  chronic stress and, 78
  depression and, 131
  interoceptive signals from, 14
generalized anxiety disorder (GAD), 119–122, 124. *See also* anxiety disorders
Gibson, Jonathan, 231
Goldin, Philippe, 83
grounding tools, 226–227
gut-brain connection, 16, 53–55, 131, 184–185
gut microbes, 54

## H

Hakomi, 7
hand over area of activation, 226
hand-to-heart (hand-to-belly) breathing, 224
Hanley, Adam, 230
Hartzell, Mary, 71
health anxiety, 59, 99, 119, 121, 123, 144, 240. *See also* anxiety disorders
heartbeat perception test, 36
hedonic control, 165
Herman, Aleksandra, 155
homeostatic control, 165
HPA (hypothalamic-pituitary-adrenal) axis, 76
hunger cues, 164
hyperarousal
  addiction and, 158–159
  definition of, 87–88
  shifting between hypoarousal and, 94–95
  symptoms of trauma, 88–92
hyperawareness, 72, 188
hypersensitivity, 50, 51, 170
hypervigilance, 64, 83, 88, 99, 113, 133, 136, 153, 158, 167, 181, 183, 214
hypoarousal
  addiction and, 159
  definition of, 88
  shifting between hyperarousal and, 94–95
  symptoms of trauma, 92–94
hyposensitivity, 50, 51, 170

## I

illness. *See also individual illnesses*
  chronic, 111
  complications from, 52–53
  psychogenic, 57
immune system
  chronic stress and, 78
  depression and, 130
  interoceptive signals from, 15
imprinting, 67
impulsivity, 155–156
insular cortex (insula), 16–17, 111, 155, 187

interoception
accessibility of, 243–244
anxiety and, 120–125
attachment and, 69–71, 74, 192
as bidirectional process, 5–6, 19–20, 49, 57
brain and, 19–20
chronic stress and, 8
complexity of, 4, 13, 22, 35, 36
definition of, 4
depression and, 134–138
emotional experience and, 23–24, 30–31
growing interest in, 7–8
history of, 4, 7–8
importance of, 29, 55, 109, 243–244
learning about, 3–4, 244
measuring, 35–46
mental health issues and, 6, 8, 28–29
mindfulness and, 229–230
physical issues and, 6, 8
problems with, 6, 8
science of, 13–22
sense of self and, 23, 25–27, 32–33, 192–193
as sensory system, 3
thinking and, 24–25, 31–32, 57–65
vagus nerve and, 15–16
interoceptive awareness
developing, 212–215, 229
forcing, 214
IBS and, 186
individual practices for enhancing, 217–227
interpersonal connections and, 191
practitioner-led approaches for enhancing, 229–241
stress and, 79–80, 179–180
interoceptive disruptions
in addiction, 154–157
chronic stress and, 8, 79–80
as common thread, 111–112, 117–118
cultural norms and, 114–115
development of, 29–34
multiple, 109
physical health and, 52–55
as spectrum, 29
synergistic impacts of, 112–115
trauma and, 86–87, 97–105
interoceptive exposure (IE), 234, 240
interoceptive messages
affective, 5
limited connection to, 30
origins of, 36
pushing through, 30
role of, 4–5, 30
sources of, 13–15
interoceptive sensitivity
definition of, 35
hyper- vs. hyposensitivity, 50, 51, 170, 174
impact of, on physical and mental health, 50–52
interoceptive walking, 225–226
interoceptors, definition of, 15
interpersonal connections
challenges with, 111, 191
in childhood and adulthood, 192, 196–197
empathy and, 193–196
interoception and, 27–28, 33–34
loneliness and, 111, 198–199
MAIA domains impacted by, 199–200
misunderstandings in, 197–198
nervous system and, 196–198
irritable bowel syndrome (IBS), 51, 53, 99, 100, 182–186, 188–189, 240

## J

James, William, 4
"June Bug" outbreak, 57

## K

Kabat-Zinn, Jon, 7, 232
Kurtz, Ron, 7

## L

Lange, Carl, 4
Levine, Peter, 7, 94, 95, 97, 234
localized body tracking, 222
loneliness, 111, 198–199
long COVID, 52, 179
longer exhale breath, 224

## M

Mahler, Kelly, 51, 170
MAIA (Multidimensional Assessment of Interoceptive Awareness) and MAIA-2
  development of, 37–38, 203
  format of, 38, 203–208
  interpreting scores on, 204, 208–212
  taking, 38
  value of, 36
MAIA domains
  addiction and, 160
  ADHD and, 176–177
  anxiety disorders and, 126–127
  autism and, 176–177
  chronic pain and, 188–189
  depression and, 138–139
  disordered eating and, 166–167
  IBS and, 188–189
  interpersonal connections and, 199–200
  migraines and, 188–189
  OCD and, 149–150
  overview of, with examples, 38–46
Marano, Giuseppe, 185
mass hysteria, 57–58
Maté, Gabor, 91
Matus, Austin, 52
MDD (major depressive disorder). *See* depression
mechanoreceptors, 15
meditation, 213–214. *See also* mindfulness
Mehling, Wolf, 38, 203, 208
mental health. *See also individual issues*
  current state of, 110
  impact of interoceptive sensitivity on, 50–52
  influence of physical health on, 179
  prediction errors and, 21–22
  role of interoception in, 6, 8, 28–29
migraines, 51, 53, 180, 182, 186–189
mindfulness
  interoception and, 229–230
  structured programs, 231–234
  trauma survivors and, 231
mindfulness-based cognitive therapy (MBCT), 7, 231, 232–233
Mindfulness-Based Stress Reduction (MBSR), 7, 231, 232
minimizing, patterns of, 59–60
movement-based practices, 224–226
Multidimensional Assessment of Interoceptive Awareness. *See* MAIA
muscle dysmorphia (MD), 141, 144–146
muscular system, 78

## N

narcissism, 33–34, 195–196
natural breath observation, 223
negative, focusing on the, 61
nervous system
  ADHD and, 173, 174–175
  autonomic, 17–19, 75–76
  coping behaviors and, 157–160
  depression and, 130, 133–134
  –informed perspective, 237
  interpersonal connections and, 196–198
  parasympathetic, 17, 77
  PTSD and, 175
  role of, 17–18
  sympathetic, 17
  trauma and, 92–93, 94–95
neurodivergence, 51–52, 169. *See also* ADHD; autism spectrum disorder
nightmares, 81, 87, 90, 235
nociceptive (pain) system, 14
nonsuicidal self-injury (NSSI), 110, 141, 146–149
not-distracting (MAIA domain)
  addiction and, 160

interpreting scores for, 209–210
OCD and, 149
overview of, with examples, 39–40
trauma and, 99
noticing (MAIA domain)
addiction and, 160
anxiety disorders and, 126–127
chronic pain and, 188
depression and, 138
IBS and, 188
interpreting scores for, 209
migraines and, 188
overview of, with examples, 38–39
trauma and, 98–99
not-worrying (MAIA domain)
anxiety disorders and, 127
chronic pain and, 189
disordered eating and, 167
IBS and, 189
interpreting scores for, 210
migraines and, 189
overview of, with examples, 40–41
trauma and, 100

## O

obsessive-compulsive disorder (OCD), 141–144, 149–150
occupational therapy, 239–240
Ogden, Pat, 236
Oldroyd, Kristina, 70, 71, 72
others
distinction between self and, 27, 28, 194–195
overidentification with, 195
overempathy, 34
overextension, 195–196
overworking, 83

## P

pain
catastrophizing, 181–182
central sensitization and, 182
chronic, 51, 61, 99, 120, 180–182, 188–189, 240
nociceptive system, 14
panic disorder, 50, 61, 63, 119–122, 240. *See also* anxiety disorders
parasympathetic nervous system (PNS), 17, 77
Pavlov, Ivan, 21
pendulation, 235
people-pleasing, 32–33
perfectionism, 83–84
physical health. *See also individual issues*
impact of interoceptive sensitivity on, 50–52
influence of mental health on, 179
interoceptive disruptions and, 52–55
role of interoception in, 6, 8, 179
positive, discounting the, 61
prediction errors, 21–22, 59–60, 62–64, 125–126, 187
predictive processing
anxiety disorders and, 125–126
cognitive distortions vs., 64–65
depression and, 131
disordered eating and, 166
migraines and, 187–188
role of, in interoception, 20–21, 62–63
premonitory urges, 143
PTSD (post-traumatic stress disorder)
alexithymia and, 101–102
attention regulation and, 101
body listening and, 103–104
definition of, 81
emotional awareness and, 101–102
history of, as official diagnosis, 85
nervous system and, 175
substance use disorders and, 123–124
symptoms of, 87–89, 101

## Q

Quadt, Lisa, 199
quick interoceptive check-in, 217–218
Quigley, Karen, 62

## R

relationships. *See* interpersonal connections
respiratory system, 13
rheumatoid arthritis, 53
Robinson, Jake, 54
rumination
  anxiety disorders and, 125
  depression and, 136–137

## S

Saltafossi, Martina, 111
SAM (sympathetic-adrenal-medullary) system, 76
Sapolsky, Robert, 75
Schore, Allan, 67, 196
self
  disrupted connection with, 148–149
  emotional experiences and, 26
  interoception and sense of, 23, 25–27, 32–33, 192–193
  narrative vs. experiential, 26
  -other distinction, 27, 28, 194–195
  trauma and loss of, 97–98
self-awareness, 26, 32
self-criticism, 83–84
self-harm. *See* nonsuicidal self-injury
self-medicating, 153
self-regulation (MAIA domain)
  addiction and, 160
  ADHD and, 177
  anxiety disorders and, 127
  autism and, 177
  interpersonal connections and, 200
  interpreting scores for, 211
  OCD and, 149–150
  overview of, with examples, 43–44
  trauma and, 102–103
sensations. *See* body sensations
Sensorimotor Psychotherapy (SP), 7, 236–237
sensory hypersensitivity, 186–187
sensory phenomena, 142–143
serotonin, 54, 130, 131, 185
Sherrington, Charles S., 4
Siegel, Daniel, 71
sitting, grounded, 227
skin-picking disorder, 141, 142–143
sleep, 78
smiling, 23
social anxiety disorder, 61, 119–121, 123, 126. *See also* anxiety disorders
social connection. *See* interpersonal connections
social media, 110, 124
somatic amplification, 100, 121, 181
Somatic Experiencing (SE), 7, 97, 234–235
somatic psychotherapy, 234
stress. *See also* chronic stress; PTSD; traumatic stress
  definition of, 80
  IBS and, 183–184
  interoceptive awareness and, 79–80, 179–180
  types of, 80–81
stressor, definition of, 77
stress response
  activation of, 75
  sequence of, 76–77
stretch-release cycles, 224–225
substance use and addiction disorders
  anxiety and, 123–124
  avoidance and, 153–154
  coping behaviors and, 153–154, 157–160
  depression and, 134, 136
  distraction and, 116, 153–154
  interoceptive disruptions and, 154–157
  MAIA domains impacted by, 160
  prevalence of, 110, 151
  trauma and, 152–153
  withdrawal, 157
suicidality, 110
Suksasilp, Chatrin, 37
sympathetic nervous system, 17

## T

tech neck, 53
technology, overuse of, 110, 111
thermoregulatory system, 14
thinking. *See also* predictive processing
cognitive distortions, 57–58, 64–65
embodied cognition, 26, 193
emotions and, 25, 60
interoception and, 24–25, 31–32, 57–65
irrational, 57–58
over-, 32
rational, 24–25, 31–32
transdiagnostic approach, 28, 111
trauma. *See also* Adverse Childhood Experiences Study; PTSD; traumatic stress
addiction and, 152–153
ADHD and, 173, 175–176
childhood, 113–114
coping behaviors and, 91–92
definition of, 80–81
disordered eating and, 162–163
effects of, 87, 95, 97
hyperarousal symptoms of, 88–92
hypoarousal symptoms of, 92–94
impacts of cumulative, 85–86
insecure attachment and, 113–114
interoceptive disruptions and, 97–105
loss of self and, 97–98
mindfulness and, 231
prevalence of, 85–86
trauma-informed yoga (TIY), 7, 237–238
traumatic stress
definition of, 80–81
interoceptive disruptions and, 86–87, 153
trust (MAIA domain)
chronic pain and, 189
depression and, 138
disordered eating and, 166–167
IBS and, 189
interpersonal connections and, 200
interpreting scores for, 212
migraines and, 189
misinterpretation of bodily sensations and, 58–59
OCD and, 149
overview of, with examples, 45–46
trauma and, 104–105

## U

urinary system, 14

## V

vagus nerve
compression of, 53
etymology of, 15
interoception and, 15–16
location of, 15–16
role of, 16
sensitization of, 53
stress and, 184
trauma and, 184
Vally, Zahir, 135–136
van der Kolk, Bessel, 86, 89, 99, 104

## W

walking, interoceptive, 225–226
weight-shifting awareness, 225
withdrawal, 157
World Health Organization (WHO), 110
worry. *See also* not-worrying; rumination
depression and, 136–137
about sensation, 61–62

## Y

yoga, trauma-informed, 7, 237–238

# Acknowledgments

This book was born through relationship—through conversations, encouragement, curiosity, and the generosity of many people who helped shape both the ideas and the process behind it. While my name appears on the cover, this work reflects a long lineage of teachers, colleagues, clients, and supporters whose influence is woven throughout these pages.

I am grateful to the organizers of TEDxChilliwack for the opportunity to speak about interoception at an event centered on clarity. Although the talk was postponed by the pandemic and ultimately recorded without an audience, the process of researching and preparing it had a lasting impact on my work. It deepened my fascination with this often-overlooked sensory system and planted the seed for a book that would later take fuller shape.

This book began with the encouragement of Tim McKee at North Atlantic Books, who reached out after watching that talk and encouraged me to write it. His curiosity about interoception—and his openness to a topic that remains unfamiliar to many—was both affirming and catalytic. I am also grateful for the patience and support of the team at North Atlantic Books, whose calm guidance helped shape a first-time author's work.

My professional appreciation extends to the teachers, researchers, and clinicians whose work has shaped my understanding of the nervous system and the mind–body connection, particularly within somatic traditions. These perspectives transformed how I understand symptoms—shifting my lens from pathology to adaptation—and continue to guide both my clinical work and my writing.

I hold deep respect and gratitude for the clients I have had the privilege of working with. Their courage, honesty, and willingness to listen inward have been my greatest teachers. While stories in this book are shared with care and privacy, the wisdom they reflect comes directly from those who trusted me with their lived experience.

I am blessed to be surrounded by family and friends who offered patience, encouragement, and steady support throughout the writing of this book. Writing can be a solitary act, but this book was sustained by connection—by those who listened, asked thoughtful questions, and reminded me why this work matters.

My deep gratitude goes to my husband, Richard—my steadfast champion and cheerleader. Thank you for your patience, the morning coffees, and for holding life together while I wrote.

Finally, I offer deepest gratitude to my Lord and Creator. We truly are "fearfully and wonderfully made." (Psalm 139:14)

# About the Author

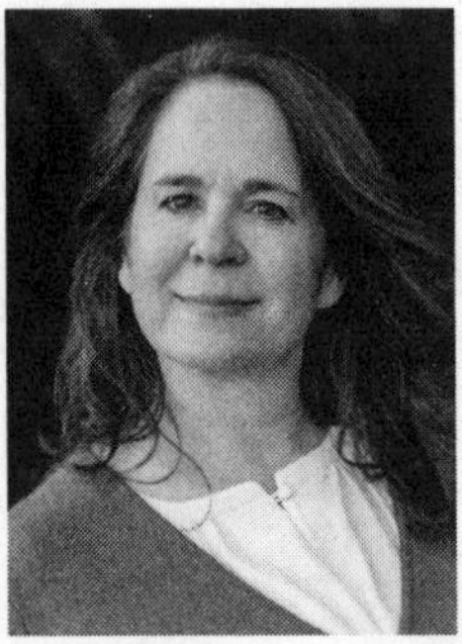

*Photo by Jen McLeod Photography*

**Carrie DeJong** is a therapist and writer with a deep curiosity about the nervous system. With nearly thirty years of clinical experience, she has dedicated her career to listening carefully, whether to stories, symptoms, or the subtle language of the body.

Carrie's work grew from a simple but powerful observation: Many people are doing everything they can to heal yet remain disconnected from the internal signals meant to guide them. Anxiety, depression, substance use, chronic stress, and trauma-related symptoms often make far more sense when viewed through the lens of an overwhelmed nervous system. This realization led her to focus on somatic approaches to trauma recovery and, ultimately, on interoception—the body's ability to sense and interpret internal experience.

Her clinical background includes trauma treatment programs for children and families, residential addiction treatment, and private practice. Drawing on neuroscience and mind–body research, Carrie helps clients rebuild trust in their bodies by learning to notice sensations, interpret them with compassion, and respond with greater choice.

An avid student of neuroscience, Carrie is particularly passionate about making complex science understandable and practical. She believes that understanding how the nervous system functions can help restore agency, reduce shame, and create space for genuine, lasting change. As an author, she writes with warmth, humility, and deep respect for the intelligence of the human body—encouraging readers to view their bodies not as problems to fix but as allies in healing.

# About North Atlantic Books

North Atlantic Books (NAB) is an independent, nonprofit publisher committed to a bold exploration of the relationships between mind, body, spirit, and nature. Founded in 1974, NAB aims to nurture a holistic view of the arts, sciences, humanities, and healing. To make a donation or to learn more about our books, authors, events, and newsletter, please visit www.northatlanticbooks.com.